CLINICAL DECISION MAKING

Case Studies for the Occupational Therapy Assistant

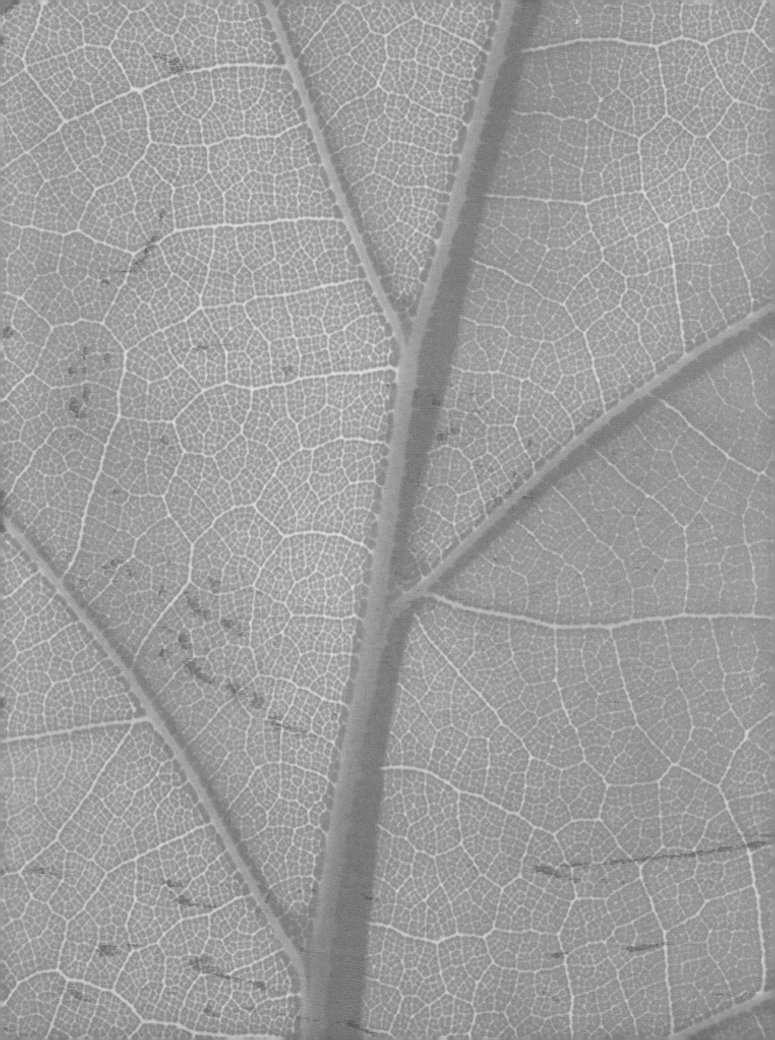

CLINICAL DECISION MAKING

Case Studies for the Occupational Therapy Assistant

Jennifer L. Theis MS, OTR/L

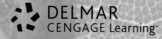

DELMAR
CENGAGE Learning™

Australia • Brazil • Japan • Korea • Mexico • Singapore • Spain • United Kingdom • United States

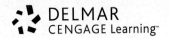

Clinical Decision Making: Case Studies for the Occupational Therapy Assistant, First Edition
Jennifer L. Theis, MS, OTR/L

Vice President, Career and Professional Editorial: Dave Garza

Director of Learning Solutions: Matthew Kane

Senior Acquisitions Editor: Sherry Dickinson

Managing Editor: Marah Bellegarde

Product Manager: Laura J. Wood

Editorial Assistant: Anthony Souza

Vice President, Career and Professional Marketing: Jennifer McAvey

Marketing Director: Wendy E. Mapstone

Marketing Coordinator: Scott A. Chrysler

Production Director: Carolyn Miller

Senior Art Director: David Arsenault

For product information and technology assistance, contact us at
Cengage Learning Customer & Sales Support, 1-800-354-9706

For permission to use material from this text or product,
submit all requests online at **cengage.com/permissions**
Further permissions questions can be emailed to
permissionrequest@cengage.com

Library of Congress Control Number: 2009942337

ISBN-13: 978-1-4354-2576-7

ISBN-10: 1-4354-2576-6

Delmar
5 Maxwell Drive
Clifton Park,
NY 12065-2919
USA

Cengage Learning is a leading provider of customized learning solutions with office locations around the globe, including Singapore, the United Kingdom, Australia, Mexico, Brazil, and Japan. Locate your local office at: **international.cengage.com/region**

Cengage Learning products are represented in Canada by Nelson Education, Ltd.

For your lifelong learning solutions, visit **delmar.cengage.com**

Visit our corporate website at **www.cengage.com**

To learn more about Delmar, visit **www.cengage.com/delmar**

Purchase any of our products at your local college store or at our preferred online store **www.CengageBrain.com**

Notice to the Reader

Publisher does not warrant or guarantee any of the products described herein or perform any independent analysis in connection with any of the product information contained herein. Publisher does not assume, and expressly disclaims, any obligation to obtain and include information other than that provided to it by the manufacturer. The reader is expressly warned to consider and adopt all safety precautions that might be indicated by the activities described herein and to avoid all potential hazards. By following the instructions contained herein, the reader willingly assumes all risks in connection with such instructions. The publisher makes no representations or warranties of any kind, including but not limited to, the warranties of fitness for particular purpose or merchantability, nor are any such representations implied with respect to the material set forth herein, and the publisher takes no responsibility with respect to such material. The publisher shall not be liable for any special, consequential, or exemplary damages resulting, in whole or part, from the readers' use of, or reliance upon, this material.

Printed in the United States of America
1 2 3 4 5 6 7 14 13 12 11 10

DEDICATION

This book is dedicated to my son Cameron and my husband Matthew Roed for their willingness to support me in expanding my professional development as an occupational therapist. I am forever indebted to them for "letting me off the hook" frequently as primary caregiver so that I could dedicate my time and mind completely to the writing and editing of this book. Without this support, I could not have completed this project.

Table of Contents

Preface   ix

About the Author   xi

Cross-Reference List   xiii

Part One **Acute Care 1**

Case Study   1   *Easy: Nancy*   3

Case Study   2   *Moderate: Clarence*   11

Case Study   3   *Difficult: Lewis*   19

Case Study   4   *Difficult: George*   27

Part Two **Skilled Nursing Facility 37**

Case Study   5   *Easy: Carolina*   39

Case Study   6   *Moderate: Clarence*   47

Case Study   7   *Difficult: George*   57

Part Three **Inpatient Rehabilitation 69**

Case Study   8   *Easy: Sandy*   71

Case Study   9   *Moderate: Stephanie*   79

Case Study 10   *Moderate: David*   89

Case Study 11   *Difficult: Isaac*   97

Case Study 12   *Difficult: George*   107

Part Four **Home Health Care 117**

Case Study 13   *Moderate: Gladys*   119

Case Study 14   *Difficult: George*   127

Part Five **Community Services 139**

Case Study 15   *Easy: Fall Prevention and Osteoporosis Screening*

at Community Center for Elderly Day Program   141

Case Study 16   *Moderate: Brian*   143

Case Study 17   *Moderate: The Autism Institute*   151

Part Six **Outpatient Rehabilitation 153**

Case Study 18   *Easy: Wendy*   155

Case Study 19   *Easy: Drivers Rehabilitation—Florence*   163

Case Study 20   *Moderate: Anupam*   173

Case Study 21   *Moderate: Hand Therapy—Brad*   183

Case Study 22   *Difficult: George*   191

Case Study 23   *Difficult: Drivers Rehabilitation—Larry*   203

Part Seven   **Federal or State Government Agencies . . 213**

Case Study 24   *Easy: Tina*   215
Case Study 25   *Difficult: Joe*   217

Part Eight   **Psychiatric Care. 227**

Case Study 26   *Moderate: Michiko*   229
Case Study 27   *Difficult: Lia*   239

General References **247**

Index. **251**

Preface

Clinical Decision Making: Case Studies for the Occupational Therapy Assistant was created for students, entry-level practitioners, and professors. It was developed as a format with which professionals can work on fostering clinical reasoning skills in the provision of occupational therapy assistant services.

This book was created because current texts for the occupational therapy assistant have limited case studies. Furthermore, the available case studies within these books are lacking in two regards: (1) incorporation of all of the settings across the continuum of care including taking a single client across this continuum and (2) incorporation of occupational therapy language as found in the Occupational Therapy Practice Framework (AOTA, 2008). The cases in this book are meant to provoke discussion about treatment planning, ethical issues, and collaboration with the client, family, and other healthcare providers.

Text Organization

The book is organized broadly using the current Occupational Therapy Practice Framework of the American Occupational Therapy Association (AOTA, 2008). Each case contains examples of how the framework can come to life in the description of a particular client. Each case includes a detailed occupational profile along with a brief summary of key points of the profile, analysis of occupational performance (e.g., current abilities and limitations in activities of daily living, instrumental activities of daily living, education, work, leisure, and social participation), factors influencing performance skills and patterns (e.g., motor, process skills, habits, routines, and roles), factors influencing contexts (e.g., cultural, social, physical, and personal), synthesis of abilities (e.g., facilitators or barriers to occupational performance), intervention plan (e.g., collaborative client-centered goals, therapeutic use of occupations and activities, consultation process, and education process), intervention review, outcomes, and discussion questions. The cases walk the reader through the most common settings in which occupational therapy assistants currently practice: (1) acute care, (2) skilled nursing facility, (3) inpatient rehabilitation, (4) home health care, (5) community services, (6) outpatient rehabilitation, (7) federal or state government agencies, and (8) psychiatric care. These cases are meant to function as a supplement to currently used texts in education of the occupational therapy assistant to foster ongoing professional development.

Road Map of How to Use the Case Studies

At the beginning of this book, the reader will find a cross-reference list highlighting (1) the level of difficulty for each case study (easy, moderate, or difficult), making it simple to grade discussions based on the skill set of the reader; (2) the area of the healthcare continuum being addressed during the specific case study (e.g., acute care, home health, federal or state government agencies); (3) the diagnosis of the client described in the individual cases; and (4) a snapshot of the primary impairments and functional deficits. To demonstrate how a client's need for occupational therapy services might change across the continuum of care, two of the clients have been described in more depth across the continuum: Clarence (Cases 2 and 6) and George (Cases 4, 7, 12, 14, and 22). The reader should make certain to check with necessary laws and practices specific to his or her state especially regarding precautions and use of modalities.

Acknowledgments

I wish to thank Rick Daniels, author of several nursing textbooks, for connecting me with Sherry Dickinson at Delmar Cengage Learning who then invited me to create these case studies. I am grateful for the guidance, feedback, and organization of project manager Laura Wood and Sini Sivaraman for keeping us on schedule. I also appreciate the efforts of reviewers and copy editors of this book, for their time and expertise in getting this book to print at its best.

A number of my colleagues in the Chicago (Illinois) and Twin Cities (Minneapolis/St. Paul, Minnesota) area, especially those at Sister Kenny Rehabilitation Institute, helped at varying levels to make these cases as realistic as possible. I would like to recognize the contributions of the following: Steve Anderson, Kerri Burrandt, Jane Fjerstad, Beth Gorman, Nicole Hoops, Brian LeLoup, Gayle Monteon, Carol Peltier, Angie Tumberg, Chris Tripp, Maureen Whitford, and Joette Zola. I am grateful for the initial ability to bounce ideas off of Nancy Flinn, an occupational therapist and former instructor for Saint Catherine's occupational therapy program. Special thanks to my mentor, Mary Vining Radomski, an occupational therapist, researcher, and co-editor of one of the leading texts for occupational therapy programs, *Occupational Therapy for Physical Dysfunction, Sixth Edition* (Radomski and Trombly Latham, eds., 2008).

Special thanks to my family for their support, because without it this book could not have been created: Caroline & Delton Roed and Larry & Sandy Theis. Thanks to my sister-in-law, Gael Orsmond, for her input on current case studies that she and her colleagues use at Boston University's occupational therapy program.

Reviewers

Delmar Cengage Learning would like to thank the following reviewers for their input and guidance throughout the development process:

Susan Cheng, MS, OTR/L
Assistant Dean, Allied Health
Program Director, OTA Program
Durham Technical Community College
Durham, North Carolina

Tammy Gipson, MS, OTR/L
OTA Program Director
Wallace State Community College
Hanceville, Alabama

Ada Boone Hoerl, MA, COTA/C
Program Coordinator and Assistant Professor
Sacramento City College
Sacramento, California

Kathi Krivanec, MA, COTA/L
OTA Program Director and Associate Professor
Briarwood College
Southington, Connecticut

Marlene Steele, COTA/C, BSHA
Instructor
Sacramento City College
Sacramento, California

About the Author

JENNIFER L. THEIS graduated from Carleton College, Northfield, Minnesota, with a Bachelor of Arts in behavioral psychology. She worked as a research technician in an orthopedic office while earning money for graduate school. She graduated from Boston University with a Master of Science degree in occupational therapy. She began her occupational therapy career in 1997 at Schwab Rehabilitation Hospital in Chicago.

In 2002, she transitioned back to the Twin Cities where she currently works as an occupational therapy practitioner, researcher, and program coordinator for the spinal cord system of care at Sister Kenny Rehabilitation Institute. She has facilitated and taught ongoing training sessions for safe transfers for therapy and nursing practitioners and students. She has also presented at national interdisciplinary conferences on her work in safe transfers.

She has contributed to occupational therapy education by creating portions of a learning DVD and PowerPoint lectures to supplement the book *Occupational Therapy for Physical Dysfunction, Sixth Edition*, edited by Mary Vining Radomski and Catherine A. Trombly Latham.

Cross-Reference List

Case		Page	Area of Practice	Level of Difficulty	Diagnosis	Primary Impairments and Functional Deficits	Related Cases
1	Nancy	3	Acute Care	Easy	Trauma to Intervertebral Disc and Vertebral Degeneration status post 3rd to 5th Lumbar (L3-L5) Fusion	Pain, general weakness, decreased mobility due to spine precautions, decreased understanding of precautions	
2	Clarence	11	Acute Care	Moderate	Congestive Heart Failure status post Coronary Artery Bypass Graft	Generalized weakness, decreased understanding of post-operative sternal precautions, decreased ability to be primary caregiver to spouse with Alzheimer's disease	6
3	Lewis	19	Acute Care	Difficult	Multiple System Failure	General weakness, minimal responsiveness, medical instability, decreased activity tolerance, diminished skin integrity, vent dependence, decreased understanding of medical condition and its impact on abilities, history of decreased healthy coping skills, inconsistent family support	
4	George	27	Acute Care	Difficult	Brain Injury and Spinal Cord Injury	Decreased medical stability, strength, coordination, mobility, sensation, energy, cognition, understanding of the effect of brain and spinal cord injuries	7, 12, 14, 22
5	Carolina	39	Skilled Nursing Facility	Easy	Osteoarthritis status post Total Knee Replacement	Pain, generalized weakness, decreased flexion and extension of knee, decreased ability to manage stairs, decreased understanding of how to incorporate knee precautions into daily activities	
6	Clarence	47	Skilled Nursing Facility	Moderate	Congestive Heart Failure status post Coronary Artery Bypass Graft	Generalized weakness, decreased understanding regarding sternal precautions, decreased ability to be primary caregiver to spouse with Alzheimer's disease	2

(Continues)

(Continued)

	Name	Setting	Difficulty	Condition	Description	References
7	George	Skilled Nursing Facility	Difficult	Brain Injury and Spinal Cord Injury	Decreased skin integrity, strength, coordination, mobility, sensation, energy, and cognition; autonomic dysreflexia and orthostatic hypotension; and decreased understanding of the effect of brain and spinal cord injuries	4, 12, 14, 22
8	Sandy	Inpatient Rehabilitation	Easy	Status post Total Hip Replacement	Pain, generalized weakness, decreased understanding of how to incorporate hip precautions into daily activities	
9	Stephanie	Inpatient Rehabilitation	Moderate	Spinal Cord Injury	Decreased strength, coordination, mobility, sensation, energy, decreased understanding of the effect of spinal cord injury	
10	David	Inpatient Rehabilitation	Moderate	Burn	Pain, decreased skin integrity, decreased range of motion, decreased ability to engage in meaningful play	
11	Isaac	Inpatient Rehabilitation	Difficult	Total Knee Replacement and Cerebrovascular Accident	Decreased balance, coordination, range of motion, comprehension, expression, cognition	
12	George	Inpatient Rehabilitation	Difficult	Brain Injury and Spinal Cord Injury	Decreased strength, coordination, mobility, sensation, energy, cognition, decreased understanding of the effect of brain and spinal cord injuries	4, 7, 14, 22
13	Gladys	Home Health Care	Moderate	Osteoporosis	Fear of falling, decreased balance, leg weakness, multiple medications, high risk of osteoporosis, limited engagement in activities	
14	George	Home Health Care	Difficult	Brain Injury and Spinal Cord Injury	Decreased strength, coordination, mobility, sensation, energy, higher-level cognition, medical stability (autonomic dysreflexia, orthostatic hypotension), and decreased understanding of the effect of brain and spinal cord injuries	4, 7, 12, 22

(Continues)

(Continued)

#	Name	Page	Setting	Difficulty	Condition	Description
15	Fall Prevention and Osteoporosis Screening at Community Center for Elderly Day Program	141	Community Services	Easy	Multiple Geriatric Clients at Risk for Falls	Presence of falls, decreased balance, decreased ability to perform timed sit to stand, decreased activity levels, fear of falling, decreased understanding of fall risk factors and prevention program
16	Brian	143	Community Services	Moderate	Autism	Decreased fine and gross motor function; decreased communication and interaction skills; decreased ability to regulate himself in response to stress and overstimulation; unwanted behaviors, including hitting head and being aggressive; and Brian, his parents, and teacher demonstrate decreased understanding of treatment options for successful inclusion in kindergarten class
17	The Autism Institute	151	Community Services	Moderate	Autism	Decreased understanding of new teachers and family members regarding autism and its treatment strategies, especially in the context of integrated elementary school classrooms
18	Wendy	155	Outpatient Rehabilitation	Easy	Guillain-Barre Syndrome	Ataxia, decreased fine motor coordination, endurance
19	Florence	163	Outpatient Rehabilitation	Easy	MD Noted Decreased Skills for Driving	Decreased reaction time, divided attention, visual processing
20	Anupam	173	Outpatient Rehabilitation	Moderate	Cerebrovascular Accident	Decreased right upper extremity strength and function, shoulder pain, headaches, fatigue, decreased higher-level cognition, ongoing decreased understanding regarding effect of personal factors and stroke
21	Brad	183	Outpatient Rehabilitation	Moderate	Peripheral Nerve Injury	Decreased sensation, decreased strength, decreased coordination, pain, decreased understanding of nerve entrapment effect on function and prevention

(Continues)

(Continued)

#	Name	Page	Setting	Title	Difficulty	Description	Cross-Reference
22	George	191	Outpatient Rehabilitation	Brain Injury and Spinal Cord Injury	Difficult	Decreased strength, coordination, mobility, sensation, energy, higher-level cognition, medical instability (autonomic dysreflexia and orthostatic hypotension), decreased understanding of the effect of brain and spinal cord injuries	4, 7, 12, 14
23	Larry	203	Outpatient Rehabilitation	Cerebrovascular Accident	Difficult	Depth perception, visual processing speed, reaction time, attention (e.g., divided, selective, and sustained), ability to follow instructions safely, ability to change lanes safely, ability to navigate intersections safely, insight into deficits	
24	Tina	215	Federal or State Government Agencies	Legal Issues of COTA Practice	Easy	Not applicable	
25	Joe	217	Federal or State Government Agencies	Major Multiple Trauma resulting in Amputation, Brain Injury, and Burn	Difficult	Decreased higher-level cognitive function, decreased military combat skills, compromised skin integrity, decreased range of motion, decreased mobility, decreased understanding regarding amputation, burns, and brain injury	
26	Michiko	229	Psychiatric Care	Bulimia Nervosa	Moderate	Poor concentration, dizziness, decreased life balance, poor life management skills, poor body image, compulsive exercising and other compensatory behaviors, decreased understanding of nutrition, stressors, and emotional reaction to food and eating	
27	Lia	239	Psychiatric Care	Paranoid Schizophrenia	Difficult	Decreased personal grooming and bathing, decreased safe child rearing, decreased performance in work and leisure, decreased communication, auditory hallucinations, thought disorganization, and paranoia	

PART ONE

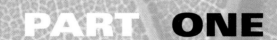

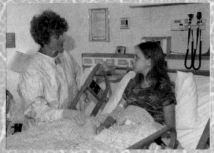

Source: Delmar/Cengage Learning.

Client and health care professional in acute care setting.

Acute Care

CASE STUDY 1

Nancy

ACUTE CARE

Level of Difficulty: Easy

Overview: Requires understanding of treatment of a working woman after back fusion in an acute care setting

Engagement in Occupation to Support Participation in Context(s)

Performance in Areas of Occupation: Full-time worker, mother, and spouse

Primary Impairments and Functional Deficits: Pain, general weakness, decreased mobility due to spine precautions, decreased understanding of precautions

Context: 45-year-old mother of two young children who works full-time in a craft store

Occupational Profile

Nancy is a 45-year-old woman who presents with sudden onset of pain, decreased strength, and sensory deficits in her legs after lifting a heavy box of supplies at work. Results of a magnetic resonance imaging (MRI) indicate damage to the intervertebral disc at the level of the 4th lumbar (L4) vertebra and mild to moderate degeneration of the vertebrae in the area. It is determined that she is a candidate for lumbar spinal fusion (L3-L5). The surgery is uncomplicated. Her impairments in strength have subsided to some degree, and she reports that the numbness has decreased.

Nancy lives with her spouse in a split-level home with four stairs and two railings up to her bedroom and bathroom. Nancy will need to manage stairs because the bedroom is on the second floor. She has access to a walk-in shower. Nancy performs the majority of the inside chores including cooking, while her spouse performs the chores outside of the house such as taking out the trash and caring for the lawn.

Nancy works full-time at a local craft store. She is responsible for helping clients, stocking shelves, and overseeing the framing section of the store. Typically, she is on her feet, standing or walking, for the entire 8-hour shift. She has two 15-minute breaks and a 30-minute lunch break.

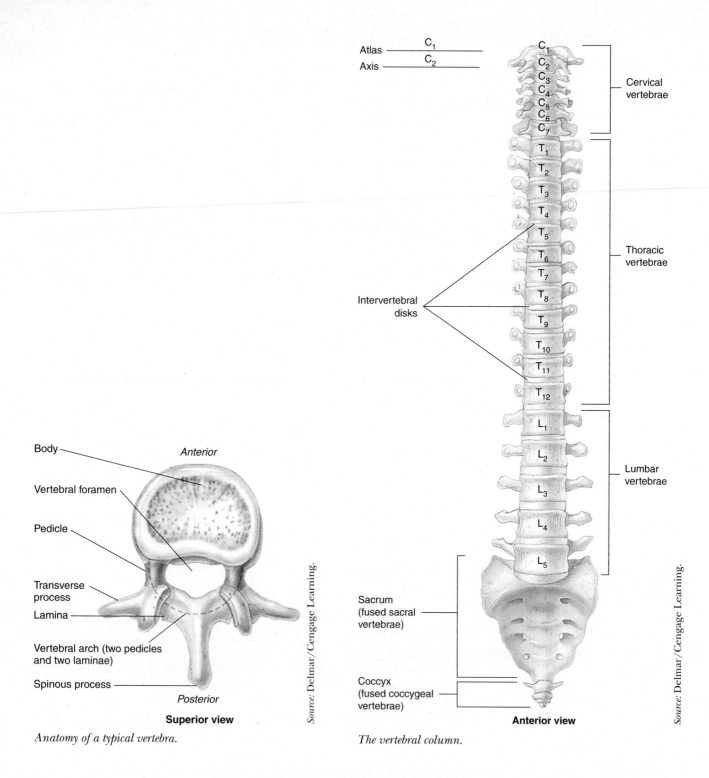

Atlas — C$_1$
Axis — C$_2$

C$_1$
C$_2$
C$_3$
C$_4$
C$_5$
C$_6$
C$_7$

Cervical vertebrae

T$_1$
T$_2$
T$_3$
T$_4$
T$_5$
T$_6$
T$_7$
T$_8$
T$_9$
T$_{10}$
T$_{11}$
T$_{12}$

Intervertebral disks

Thoracic vertebrae

L$_1$
L$_2$
L$_3$
L$_4$
L$_5$

Lumbar vertebrae

Sacrum (fused sacral vertebrae)

Coccyx (fused coccygeal vertebrae)

Anterior view

Source: Delmar/Cengage Learning.

The vertebral column.

Body
Vertebral foramen
Pedicle
Transverse process
Lamina
Vertebral arch (two pedicles and two laminae)
Spinous process

Anterior

Posterior

Superior view

Source: Delmar/Cengage Learning.

Anatomy of a typical vertebra.

Nancy and her spouse have two children under the age of 8. Nancy is active in her children's Parent Teacher Association.

Nancy is one-day post spine surgery. She has been seen for one session of physical therapy (PT) and the practitioner recommended consultation with occupational therapy (OT). She is an excellent candidate for 1 to 3 sessions of OT within the acute care setting. The primary physician has ordered consults for OT, PT, case management (CM), nursing, and surgical and internal medicine physicians.

**Analysis of
Occupational
Performance**

Synthesis of Occupational Profile

Nancy is a 45-year-old married woman status post fusion of her L3-L5 vertebrae. She is a spouse, mother, and full-time worker in a craft store. She presents for OT within the acute care setting to address decreased understanding of spine precautions, potential equipment needs, and occupational training in the areas of lower body dressing, toileting, bathing, stair management, light home management, and eventual return to work in an effort to resume her previous occupational roles.

Observed Performance in Desired Occupation/Activity

Activities of Daily Living

Bathing: Nancy requires moderate assistance to complete bathing. She is able to wash her upper body, but needs assistance to wash her right lower leg, foot, and bottom. Nancy needs help to cover her incision. Her surgeon has recommended that she stand for the entire shower to protect her spinal fusion. She needs to transfer in and out of the shower with her brace on, but then she may take it off to shower completely.

Dressing: Nancy is able to put on her own shirt, but she cannot don or doff her thoracolumbosacral orthosis (TLSO). She requires maximal assistance for lower body dressing. Nancy is not able to cross her legs yet without bending or twisting her spine or experiencing pain. After someone helps her initiate donning her underwear and pants, she is able to stand up with minimal assistance to start to pull the clothes up the rest of the way except for requiring help to get them over her bottom and the TLSO. She is unable to put on her socks or her shoes.

Functional Mobility: She requires minimal assistance for her functional mobility. She needs help to get up into standing, but she is then able to walk for short distances (i.e., less than 150 feet) without any assistive device and supervision.

Sexual Activity: Nancy is interested in understanding any limitations to her sexual activity related to her spine precautions.

Sleep/Rest: As a result of the surgery, Nancy is less able to get comfortable throughout the night. Her sleep has been interrupted. She also finds that she needs to sleep during the day secondary to pain and fatigue; she did not need to do this prior to the injury.

Toileting: Nancy requires maximum assistance with toileting. She is able to get her clothing down before going to the bathroom, but she needs help to get them back up. She is unable to wipe herself without laterally bending or twisting her spine.

Instrumental Activities of Daily Living

Child Rearing: Nancy has two daughters under the age of 8. She is the primary caregiver and gets both children ready for school. She is home from work in time to get them from the school bus in the afternoon.

Community Mobility: Since her surgery, Nancy has not attempted community mobility. She drove before her surgery and is interested in learning about any driving restrictions.

Health Management and Maintenance: Outside of this new spine injury, Nancy has been relatively healthy. She goes to her doctor for annual check-ups. The only medication she takes is pain reliever, which she needed once her back pain became unbearable.

Home Establishment and Management; Meal Preparation and Cleanup: Nancy is responsible for the cooking and cleaning at home. Her spouse helps with some of the heavier cleaning, taking out the trash, and taking care of the lawn.

Shopping: Nancy is responsible for shopping, especially groceries. On Sundays she typically drives herself to the grocery store.

Education

Formal Educational Participation: Nancy completed high school. She did not pursue further education, so that she could start a family and work.

Work

Job Performance: As stated before, Nancy works full-time at a local craft store. She is responsible for helping clients, stocking shelves, and overseeing the framing section of the store.

Retirement Preparation and Adjustment: Nancy is not ready to retire soon. If she is unable to handle the essential job functions at the craft store, she may need to explore changing jobs or job retraining because she and her spouse cannot afford to lose her income.

Leisure

Leisure Participation: Nancy has limited time to perform any leisure activities. She spends her time going to her children's sporting and dance events.

Social Participation

Community: Nancy is active in her children's school through the Parent Teacher Association.

Family: Nancy is married with two children under the age of 8. Her spouse is supportive, but he works full-time and cannot take time off from work to help her.

Peer, Friend: Nancy has several friends in the area, but she has spent most of her time with her family or at work.

Factors Influencing Performance Skills and Patterns

Motor Skills

Mobility: Pain and mild general weakness decreased Nancy's mobility. She has recently been able to get up to stand and walk briefly with the physical therapist in acute care without any assistive device and with minimal assistance.

Strength and Effort: Despite her pain with certain movements, Nancy's strength is 4+/5 throughout her upper and lower extremities.

Energy: Due to pain, Nancy's mobility has been more limited than usual. She has become generally weakened and has lower energy levels compared to usual.

Process Skills

Knowledge: Nancy has a basic understanding of body mechanics, but she is not able to state her spine precautions and how to incorporate them consistently into tasks such as lower body dressing, bathing, toileting, or her work at the craft store.

Habits and Routines

Nancy's morning and evening routines related to lower body dressing, bathing, toileting, meal preparation, and home management have been disrupted because of the need to incorporate her spine precautions.

Roles

Nancy is currently unable to return to work until she is able to ambulate 500 feet on unlevel surfaces, stand for over 30 minutes consecutively, and lift at least 20 pounds.

Factors Influencing Context(s)

Cultural

Nancy is Caucasian. She has a strong work ethic and she values her family.

Physical

Nancy has to deal with a split-level home along with a work setting that demands moderate lifting.

Social

Nancy and her spouse enjoy socializing with their friends. She has a supportive family although her spouse works full-time and is only available to help if needed on weekends or in the evening.

Personal

Nancy is a 45-year-old woman who works full-time in a craft store.

Synthesis of Abilities and Deficits

Facilitators to Occupational Performance

Nancy has a general knowledge of body mechanics and back care. She has been in good general health in spite of the injury to her lumbar spine. She demonstrates good strength and motivation. Nancy's family is able to provide help if needed on the weekends or evenings.

Barriers to Occupational Performance

Nancy has pain and mild general weakness that limit her independence. She needs to wear a TLSO brace and needs to be able to manage this independently because her spouse works full-time. Although she understands general body mechanics, she demonstrates a limited understanding regarding how to adhere to spine precautions during her daily routine. Nancy needs to be able to ambulate 500 feet on unlevel surfaces, stand for over 30 minutes consecutively, and lift at least 20 pounds to be able to return to work.

Intervention

Intervention Plan

Collaborative Client Goals That Are Objective and Measurable

Nancy has an anticipated duration of treatment 3-5 days, with an estimated frequency of 1-3 treatment sessions. By the time of discharge, Nancy will perform the following:

1. Donning and doffing TLSO independently with good adherence to spine precautions
2. Lower body dressing with modified independence and adaptive equipment as needed
3. Toileting with modified independence and equipment as needed
4. Bathing with modified independence and appropriate adaptive and durable medical equipment as needed
5. Incorporating a good understanding of spine precautions during daily routine, including light home management (i.e., making a bed and simple meal preparation)

By the time of discharge, Nancy's family will perform the following:

1. Demonstrating good understanding of equipment and assistance needs for discharge

Discharge Needs and Plan

Nancy is planning to return home. She needs to be able to learn how to incorporate spine precautions into her daily routine. She needs to be able to manage stairs to get to her bedroom and bathroom. Depending on her flexibility and ability to maintain her spine precautions, she may need to buy adaptive and durable medical equipment before discharge. Nancy's spouse is available to help only at night and during the weekends because of his work, so Nancy will need to be independent. In case she needs assistance with bathing, Nancy's spouse will still benefit from education and training. It is anticipated that after leaving the acute care setting of the hospital, she will not need any further OT.

Intervention Implementation

Therapeutic Use of Occupations and Activities

Occupation-Based Activities

Lower body dressing

Bathing/showering

Light home management

Work

Mobility

    Bed mobility with log rolling

Purposeful Activities

Practice putting on socks with or without equipment while maintaining spine precautions

Practice putting on underwear and pants with or without equipment while maintaining spine precautions

Practice unmaking and making a bed

Practice transferring on and off various surfaces (e.g., bed, shower, toilet, car)

Preparatory Methods

Physical agent modalities: ice

Consultation Process

Collaborating to determine equipment needs for safest lower body dressing and bathing

Collaborating to determine safe bathing options

Education Process

Training client and family about equipment recommendations.

Providing education of spine precautions during daily activities

Recommending work site modifications for return to work

Intervention Review

Daily informal meetings set with OT to review progress, review treatment plan, and make modifications as needed.

Outcomes   Besides reviewing progress toward Nancy's objective goals, therapy will focus on her ability to resume participation in her roles as full-time worker, spouse, and mother.

Questions

1. After clarification with the surgeon's office, you find out that Nancy is able to put her TLSO brace on when sitting up. She is also able to have it off when showering. Nancy is able to get the shell of the brace on and off with increased time and occasional cues to avoid twisting. However, she is unable to reach the Velcro straps that are on the back of the brace. Nancy's spouse is unable to help with managing the brace due to working full-time. What might be your options for making certain that Nancy can manage the brace herself?

2. When Nancy goes to the bathroom, you notice that she cannot reach to wipe herself after a bowel movement, what might you suggest to improve independence?

3. What discussion might you have regarding Nancy's work situation and helping to prepare for return to work?

4. What would be some home modifications that would be helpful for Nancy to avoid bending, lifting, and twisting her lumbar spine during her daily routine?

5. What would be some changes to Nancy's abilities that might affect the decision that Nancy is safe to return home at a modified independent level for the majority of the day?

6. You plan to do a shower with Nancy for your treatment session. After you remove the dressing over the incision, you notice the following: drainage, redness, shininess, and the skin around the incision is warm to touch. What do you do next?

ACUTE CARE

Level of Difficulty: Moderate

Overview: Requires understanding of treatment of an elderly person in an acute care setting after coronary artery bypass graft who is primary caregiver to his spouse who has Alzheimer's disease

Engagement in Occupation to Support Participation in Context(s)

Performance in Areas of Occupation: Spouse and primary caregiver, father, grandfather, active church member, and church choir member

Primary Impairments and Functional Deficits: Generalized weakness, decreased understanding of post-operative sternal precautions, decreased ability to be primary caregiver to spouse with Alzheimer's disease

Context: Elderly married Caucasian man who is primary caregiver of spouse with Alzheimer's disease

Occupational Profile

Clarence is an 85-year-old married man status post triple coronary artery bypass graft (CABG). Initially, Clarence experienced chest pain radiating down into his left upper extremity. He was admitted to the emergency room and found to have a myocardial infarction as a result of three blocked coronary arteries. It was determined that he would undergo emergency coronary artery bypass grafting. He tolerated the surgery with minimal complications other than difficulties with hypotension.

Clarence has been married for almost 65 years to his spouse, Adelaide. They have four grown sons, two of whom live in the nearby area. The sons and their families have been helping out with heavier chores around the house, grocery shopping, finances, and preparing meals that Clarence can reheat in the microwave. Clarence's spouse has Alzheimer's disease and he has been her primary caregiver for the past 15 years.

Clarence and Adelaide live in an apartment in the independent living center of a senior building. They have a tub/shower combo, small kitchen with a gas oven and stove, two bedrooms, and a living room. The bathroom is accessible with grab bars by the toilet and tub/shower.

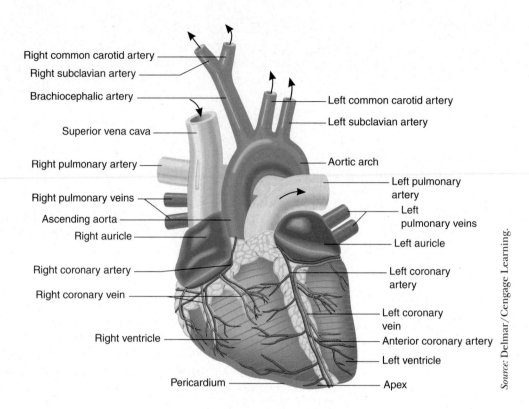

Right common carotid artery

Right subclavian artery

Brachiocephalic artery

Superior vena cava

Right pulmonary artery

Right pulmonary veins

Ascending aorta

Right auricle

Right coronary artery

Right coronary vein

Right ventricle

Left common carotid artery

Left subclavian artery

Aortic arch

Left pulmonary artery

Left pulmonary veins

Left auricle

Left coronary artery

Left coronary vein

Anterior coronary artery

Left ventricle

Pericardium

Apex

Anterior view of the heart.

Source: Delmar/Cengage Learning.

Every week, Clarence and his spouse actively attend church, where Clarence sings in the choir. Clarence drives both to church and to various other areas around town. He just renewed his license and successfully passed a defensive driving course.

Clarence is two days post CABG. He has been cleared for activity but remains on telemetry monitoring. The doctor in acute care has ordered both OT and PT services. Additional ordered services include CM, nursing, and surgical and internal medicine physicians.

Analysis of Occupational Performance

Synthesis of Occupational Profile

Clarence is an 85-year-old married man with recent coronary bypass graft secondary to blocked coronary arteries that resulted in a heart attack. He is the primary caregiver for his spouse, who has Alzheimer's disease. Clarence is also a father, grandfather, and active church member. He presents to OT within the acute care hospital setting to address difficulties with sit to stand, dressing, washing, toileting, home management, overall general weakness, and sternal precautions.

Observed Performance in Desired Occupation/Activity

Activities of Daily Living

Bathing: He requires maximum assistance for bathing; Clarence is able to wash his upper body by himself except for needing assistance to wash his incision site properly to prevent infections. He is unable to wash his lower body independently without violating his sternal precautions. Due to his compromised balance, he needs to maintain hold of a grab bar during the entire shower, and midway through needs to sit on a chair secondary to fatigue. By the end of the shower he is extremely fatigued.

Bowel and Bladder Management: To avoid straining, Clarence is on bowel medications. Additionally he is having difficulty with urinary retention after removal of the Foley catheter, so he needs to have a bladder scan each time after he voids. A few times, the nurses have had to perform straight catheterization due to evidence of retention of residual urine on the bladder ultrasound.

Dressing: Clarence requires supervision for upper body dressing due to his need for assistance with setup to obtain his clothes; Clarence is able to put on both a pullover shirt and a button-down shirt by himself. Despite his ability to do so independently, it is evident that he requires increased time. Clarence requires maximum assistance for lower body dressing; Clarence needs help to start donning his underwear and pants, but after getting minimal assistance to stand he is able to pull them up over his hips and bottom himself. He is dependent in donning his compression garments and shoes at this time.

Functional Mobility: He requires moderate assistance to complete his functional mobility overall. He is able to roll to both sides when in bed while maintaining his sternal precautions, but he needs help to get from his side up into sitting. Owing to generalized weakness, Clarence is having difficulty standing up from sitting by himself. However, after getting up, he is able to walk 50-75 feet supervised without any assistive device. Clarence benefits from holding a pillow across his chest to help remember his sternal precautions and to protect the incision during exertion. He also uses the pillow when coughing or sneezing to limit pain.

Sexual Activity: In spite of Adelaide's dementia, Clarence and his spouse have kept a relatively active level of intimacy. Clarence is concerned how his heart surgery will affect their intimacy and whether he should be worried about another myocardial infarction while they are having sex.

Sleep/Rest: Clarence reports that he has been sleeping better in the hospital than he does at home because he does not have to be concerned about Adelaide's wandering/safety.

Toileting: Clarence requires maximum assistance to complete his toileting tasks. He is able to pull down his pants and underwear and then sits down to urinate or defecate. He needs help to wipe himself after a bowel movement because of fear of hurting his chest. When able to urinate, Clarence can perform his own personal hygiene without assistance. Clarence requires moderate assist to get up from sitting into standing, but he can then pull up his clothes with standby assistance.

Instrumental Activities of Daily Living

Care of Others: As stated before, Clarence has been the primary caregiver for his spouse Adelaide for the past 15 years. As her dementia has progressed, he has needed to help her more and has taken over most of the responsibilities around the house.

Community Mobility: Clarence drove before this hospital admission. He recently successfully passed a defensive driving course when he renewed his license. Clarence's sons have stated that they are willing to help drive their parents to church and medical appointments including follow-up cardiac rehabilitation as needed until his sternal precautions are discontinued and Clarence is able to resume driving.

Financial Management: As care of Adelaide increased, Clarence relinquished control of his finances to his eldest son, who is a tax accountant.

Health Management and Maintenance: Prior to admission, Clarence went to his doctor for annual physicals. He was independent with managing his medications for hypertension, anticoagulation, hypercholesterolemia, and congestive heart failure. After Clarence's bypass surgery, his cardiologist is changing some of the dosages of his previous medications as well as adding new ones.

Home Establishment and Management; Meal Preparation and Cleanup: Clarence was in charge of all areas regarding home management and meal preparation, although his children would bring frozen meals that he could reheat as needed. Currently, Clarence is unable to perform any of these chores/tasks because of decreased endurance. He needs to learn how to change his diet and his spouse's to account for cardiac concerns, particularly related to decreasing cholesterol, fat, and sodium intake.

Safety Procedures and Emergency Responses: Clarence is aware of safety and emergency procedures related to his and his wife's health. While in the hospital, he has attempted to get up by himself at night to go to the bathroom even though he cannot get up without compromising his sternal precautions.

Shopping: Clarence gets help from his sons and their families for the majority of shopping needs.

Education

Formal Educational Participation: Clarence has a high school education.

Work

Retirement Preparation and Adjustment: Clarence is a retired insurance salesman. Although he saved well for his retirement, he and Adelaide are on a fixed income.

Leisure

Leisure Participation: Clarence enjoys getting together with other people in their senior building. The center offers various events that he tries to attend in spite of increasing care for Adelaide. Clarence used to enjoy playing cribbage and bridge, but has not been playing either game because of taking care of Adelaide.

Social Participation

Community: Clarence is heavily involved in his church as an elder and a choir member. Additionally, he tries to remain active with others in their senior building.

Family: As stated before, Clarence has a strong commitment to his marriage and taking care of his spouse, Adelaide, who has Alzheimer's disease. His family is supportive of both him and his spouse, particularly the two sons who live nearby.

Peer, Friend: Clarence spends time as able with friends in the building for seniors, but this has been less frequent because of the increased amount of time caring for Adelaide.

Factors Influencing Performance Skills and Patterns

Motor Skills

Mobility: Clarence is having the most difficulty with getting up from lying on his side into sitting and from sitting into standing; he requires moderate assistance for both of these tasks. He benefits from elevated surfaces such as a higher bed or a raised toilet seat to facilitate coming to stand. Once standing, he is able to ambulate 50-75 feet with standby assistance without use of any assistive device on level surfaces. Clarence ambulates slowly to make sure that he does not lose his balance and because he gets short of breath when walking faster.

Strength and Effort: Clarence is generally weak all over. His overall strength is 4-/5 throughout both his upper and lower extremities except for his quadriceps and gluteus, which are 3/5.

Energy: Clarence fatigues easily with most activities, requiring frequent rest breaks. His overall endurance is poor to fair minus. He is able to engage in an activity for only 3 to 5 minutes before needing to take a rest. During 30 minutes of activity, he takes at least 15 rest breaks. He needs to rest for at least 3 minutes before resuming. Clarence is unable to sing a hymn due to decreased cardiorespiratory status.

Process Skills

Knowledge: Clarence is knowledgeable about his previous cardiac issues regarding medication management. However, he demonstrates decreased understanding of modifications to his medication routine, comprehensive understanding of his sternal precautions, and cardiac diet restrictions that will need to be instituted at home.

Habits and Routines

Clarence's daily routine of getting dressing, bathing, toileting, and taking care of his spouse has been disrupted since the surgery.

Roles

Clarence is a spouse and caregiver, father, grandfather, and active church member. His CABG surgery and sternal precautions have disrupted his role as caregiver to his wife Adelaide. Furthermore, in order to take part in the church choir Clarence will need to have one of his sons drive him to church until his sternal precautions are discontinued and he is able to resume driving.

Factors Influencing Context(s)

Cultural

Clarence is Caucasian. He values his family and his Christian background. He attends church every Sunday and sings in the choir.

Physical

Clarence's primary physical barriers are related to difficulty getting up from lying on his side and standing up from sitting on lower surfaces. It may be necessary for various surfaces at home to be elevated to increase Clarence's adherence to his precautions.

Social

Clarence prides himself in being extremely active socially, although this has been more limited as taking care of Adelaide's needs has increased. His friends in the building for seniors are very supportive as far as offering help and checking in to make sure that Clarence and Adelaide are doing well.

Personal

Clarence is an 85-year-old married man who is the primary caregiver for his spouse.

Synthesis of Abilities and Deficits

Facilitators to Occupational Performance

Clarence is cognitively intact. His sons are supportive and have been helping with heavier home management tasks, finances, and errands. Clarence recently passed a defensive driving test and has a current driving license. Before his myocardial infarction and subsequent surgery, Clarence maintained his health fairly well in spite of cardiac issues. Clarence remains active with his church, especially the choir.

Barriers to Occupational Performance

Clarence is generally weakened not only from his myocardial infarction and surgery, but also from a long history of cardiac problems. Although he has tried to manage his health well, he has not understood how to incorporate a cardiac diet into the meals that he prepares for himself and Adelaide. She has late-stage Alzheimer's disease and is unable to provide assistance or supervision. Furthermore, Clarence has been and continues to be Adelaide's primary caregiver.

Intervention

Intervention Plan

Collaborative Client Goals That Are Objective and Measurable

Clarence has an anticipated duration of treatment 5-7 days, with an estimated frequency of 3-5 treatment sessions. By the time of discharge, Clarence will perform the following:

1. Functional transfers (sit to stand, toilet, tub/shower, car, bed) with supervision from elevated surfaces as needed
2. Bathing with minimal assistance with appropriate adaptive equipment as needed
3. Lower body dressing with supervision and good adherence to post-operative sternal precautions
4. Toileting with supervision using appropriate equipment

5. Consistent understanding and incorporation of sternal precautions during daily routine

6. Consistent understanding and ideas for incorporation of cardiac diet for meal planning at home

Discharge Needs and Plan

Clarence is planning to return home. He needs to be extremely independent because his spouse has Alzheimer's disease. His children can help with running errands and setting up meals, but they cannot provide consistent assistance and supervision. It is anticipated that after leaving the acute care hospital setting, Clarence will benefit from either transitioning to a skilled nursing facility or an inpatient rehabilitation unit.

Intervention Implementation

Therapeutic Use of Occupations and Activities

Occupation-Based Activities

Dressing

Bathing/showering

Sexual activity

Care of others

Home management

Health management and maintenance
Medication management

Financial management

Mobility
Bed mobility with log rolling with arms crossed
Sit to stand with arms crossed

Purposeful Activities

Practice putting on socks with or without equipment while maintaining sternal precautions

Practice putting on underwear and pants with or without equipment while maintaining sternal precautions

Practice unmaking and making a bed

Practice getting on and off of various surfaces (e.g., bed, toilet, tub/shower, car) while maintaining sternal precautions

Practice setting up medications for the week

Make one or two items for meal using recipes from Cardiac Diet Cookbook

Preparatory Methods

Physical agent modalities: ice

Cardiac calisthenics

Exercises

Consultation Process

Collaborating to determine the following:

Safest equipment needs for dressing, toileting, and bathing

Safe bathing options

Education Process

Client and family training of equipment use and supervision/assistance recommendations

Providing education regarding incorporation of sternal precautions during daily activities

Intervention Review

Daily informal meetings set with OT to review progress, review treatment plan, and make modifications as needed.

Outcomes

In addition to reviewing Clarence's progress toward his objective goals, therapy will focus on his ability to resume participation in his roles as spouse and primary caregiver, father, and active church member.

Questions

1. What are some essential questions that would help guide discharge planning for Clarence?

2. An important part of rehabilitation within the acute care setting for Clarence would be to determine whether his home setup fits his recommended activity level. Because of caring for his spouse, Clarence may need to be able to do more activities as compared to someone else his age. How would this affect your treatment sessions with Clarence?

3. How might the treatment and discharge plans be affected if Clarence had bariatric needs?

4. How would the treatment and discharge plans be affected if Clarence were also diabetic?

5. How would the treatment and discharge plans be affected if Clarence demonstrated significant cognitive deficits?

6. What would a treatment session for showering/bathing be focused on for Clarence?

7. Clarence reports that in the middle of the night he had to get up to go to the bathroom urgently. The nursing aide pulled on his shoulder to help him out of bed, and now Clarence reports a clicking at his chest. What should you suspect? What should you do?

8. What would your family training sessions be focused on? Whom would you involve?

9. Pick an activity that Clarence typically performs and show how to break the activity down into parts that he can perform to build up his activity tolerance.

Lewis

Level of Difficulty: Difficult

Overview: Requires understanding of treatment of an American Indian adult with multiple system failure in an intensive care unit within the acute care setting of a hospital

Engagement in Occupation to Support Participation in Context(s)

Performance in Areas of Occupation: Brother, uncle, friend, and American Indian community center member

Primary Impairments and Functional Deficits: General weakness, minimal responsiveness, medical instability, decreased activity tolerance, diminished skin integrity, vent dependence, decreased understanding of medical condition and its impact on abilities, history of decreased healthy coping skills, inconsistent family support

Context: 35-year-old unemployed American Indian man

Occupational Profile

Lewis is a 35-year-old right-handed American Indian man who presented to the emergency department with a scrotal abscess that had become septic. While in the emergency department, Lewis went into multi-system failure. The sepsis led to a cascade of medical events, finally including the need for mechanical respiratory ventilation and surgery to manage the spreading infection from the scrotal abscess.

At the time when Lewis required mechanical ventilation, he medically stabilized, but he is now in the intensive care unit (ICU) with close monitoring. Lewis has a complicated past medical history, including the original scrotal abscess. He has a long history of substance abuse, primarily alcohol and marijuana. He has gone through several chemical dependency treatment programs but continues to have difficulty with maintaining sobriety. His recurrent chemical abuse has resulted in cirrhosis of his liver. For a long time he has battled issues with weight, and he falls into the morbidly obese category.

Lewis has a nasogastric (NG) tube for feeding, along with receiving parenteral nutrition because of an inability to manage adequate safe protein intake through the feeding tube. He also is hooked up to cardiac telemetry monitors to alert medical staff to arrhythmias and other heart problems (e.g., blood pressure, heart rate, pulse oximetry), and he has arterial lines to measure his carbon dioxide levels, drainage tubes from packed wounds, a fecal tube, and a Foley catheter.

Lewis's family history is difficult to obtain, but apparently he lives with his sister's family on a reservation and provides occasional babysitting for his sister's children. Lewis is the primary caregiver for the family dog. Lewis's mother recently died from cirrhosis of the liver.

In the past, he had worked a variety of odd jobs to make ends meet. He is currently unemployed and has had difficulty keeping a steady job. Lewis receives a small stipend from the government because of his American Indian heritage.

He is an ideal candidate for 1-2 sessions per week of OT while in the intensive care unit of the acute care hospital. The primary physician has ordered consults from OT, PT, speech language pathology (SLP), CM, nursing, and surgical and internal medicine physicians.

Analysis of Occupational Performance

Synthesis of Occupational Profile

Lewis is a 35-year-old unemployed, right-handed American Indian man who went into multi-system failure due to sepsis from a scrotal abscess. He has a long history of chemical dependency, which has resulted in cirrhosis of the liver. He is also morbidly obese. Currently, he is minimally responsive and is dependent for all of his daily cares. He lives with his sister and her family, and they would like to bring him home once he is medically stable. He is now in the ICU and is being seen by OT to facilitate increased responsiveness, maintain range of motion (ROM) and proper positioning, and provide family training.

Observed Performance in Desired Occupation/Activity

Activities of Daily Living

Bathing: Lewis is dependent for bathing. He is washed via a sponge bath and is unable to help.

Bowel and Bladder Management: He is dependent for his bowel and bladder management. Lewis has a fecal tube and an indwelling Foley catheter. He is unable to control either his bowel or bladder. These tubes were inserted to protect him from integumentary system issues and potential spread of sepsis.

Dressing: Lewis is dependent for total-body dressing, and two caregivers are necessary to get Lewis dressed. Because he has so many tubes and other medical devices, he wears a hospital gown.

Eating and Feeding: He is dependent for eating. Because of his low level of responsiveness, he was on a nasogastric (NG) tube for protein supplements, but after he vomited during a respiratory therapy treatment he was converted to receiving total parenteral nutrition.

Functional Mobility: Lewis is dependent for his overall functional mobility. He is unable to help support his body when being moved. The nurses have been repositioning him using an overhead ceiling lift; alternatively, moving him requires the complete physical assistance of three staff members. He can be lifted over into a tilt-in-space manual wheelchair. Once in the wheelchair, he can sit up for 30 minutes, but then his vital signs change (e.g., hypotension, decreased oxygen saturation).

Personal Grooming: He requires total assistance to complete grooming. Lewis opens his eyes when his face is being washed or shaved, but he inconsistently turns his head to make eye contact with his caregivers.

Sexual Activity: Presently this is unknown because of Lewis's level of responsiveness.

Sleep/Rest: Lewis is able to open his eyes in response to his name or a sternal rub. He is able to keep his eyes open for about 1 minute before shutting them again.

Toileting: He is dependent for all toileting; Lewis currently has a fecal tube and indwelling Foley catheter.

Instrumental Activities of Daily Living

Community Mobility: He is dependent for his mobility within the community; this is not a core area to be worked on at this time, because of his level of abilities and medical stability.

Health Management and Maintenance: Based on the available information in the medical chart, Lewis appears to have had a chronic history of struggling with the effects of alcohol abuse/dependency.

Finances: According to his family, Lewis has had difficulty with finances, especially because he has been unable to hold a steady job.

Education

Formal Educational Participation: Lewis dropped out of high school when he was 16. He was found to have a learning disability, but even with help at school did not like to participate in traditional structured schooling.

Work

Job Performance: Lewis is currently unemployed. He has had difficulty holding a steady job. To attempt to make ends meet he has done a variety of odd jobs. He babysits his sister's children as a way to help out around the home.

Leisure

Leisure Participation: Lewis is unable to state his interests, but his sister has said that he enjoys computer games. He also loves learning anything to do with his American Indian background, including making dream catchers.

Social Participation

Community: Lewis is active with the American Indian community center.

Family: Lewis lives with his sister's family. They are supportive although frustrated by his ongoing struggles with substance abuse. According to his sister, Lewis has been severely affected by the death of their mother.

Peer, Friend: Although Lewis has a number of friends; they also have issues with substance abuse and have contributed to his ongoing difficulties remaining sober.

Factors Influencing Performance Skills and Patterns

Motor Skills

Mobility: As stated before, Lewis is unable to move without the assistance of three caregivers or an overhead ceiling lift. He can tolerate being upright in a tilt-in-space wheelchair for up to but no longer than 30 minutes.

Strength and Effort: Because Lewis is only minimally responsive, determining his overall strength is difficult. He does move all of his extremities around at times, but not in response to any commands. He is able to open his eyes inconsistently to his name for about a minute and then he closes them.

Energy: Lewis's energy is poor, with changes in his vital signs such as increased hypotension and decreased oxygen saturation noted after less than 30 minutes of sitting upright.

Respiratory Function

As Lewis became more septic his respiratory status became compromised. He was intubated and then extubated a few days later. He now is dependent on a ventilator for his breathing because of his minimally responsive state and ongoing issues with compromised respiratory capacity.

Sensation

Lewis's sensory awareness is difficult to determine because of his limited, localized responses.

Skin Characteristics

Vascularity: Areas surrounding the original scrotal abscess have opened, but the area has good vascular characteristics with no evidence of necrotic tissue.

Surface Appearance: The skin is wet with evidence of tunneling at some of the edges of the wound bed.

Swelling: There continues to be inflammation and swelling at and surrounding the scrotal abscess site.

Height: The overall wound area measures 2 by 3 centimeters.

Pigmentation: Overall, the pigmentation remains unchanged except for signs of erythema directly over the original scrotal abscess.

Process Skills

Knowledge: Because he is minimally responsive, it is difficult to ascertain Lewis's level of knowledge. His sister and her family demonstrate a decreased understanding of his medical condition and the potential magnitude of the caregiving situation upon discharge to home.

Habits and Routines

Lewis's habits and routines have been interrupted completely. At present, he and his caregivers are working on the following: achieving and maintaining medical stability, achieving optimal wound healing, and progressing his level of arousal/responsiveness including being able to establish a functional means of communication.

Roles

Lewis is a brother, uncle, friend, and an American Indian community center member.

Factors Influencing Context(s)

Cultural

Lewis is an American Indian and his culture is incredibly important to him. He tries to be active in his local community center.

Physical

The family home has multiple steps with no rails to enter. Once in the home, there is an additional flight of stairs with one railing to get up to Lewis's bedroom and bathroom. The tub in the bathroom is an old-fashioned one with claw feet. To live on only one level in the family home would be difficult for Lewis.

Social

Lewis's family and the community center provide the bulk of his social support. His friends are not very supportive and have contributed to his ongoing involvement in substance abuse.

Personal

Lewis is a 35-year-old unemployed American Indian man.

Synthesis of Abilities and Deficits

Facilitators to Occupational Performance

Lewis has strong support from his family and American Indian community center. He is beginning to show signs of increased responsiveness such as opening his eyes when his name is called, he is moved or sat up, or his face is washed. He has a strong connection and interest in his American Indian heritage.

Barriers to Occupational Performance

Lewis has had numerous medical complications and is still not medically stable. Lewis is minimally responsive with limited ability to interact with his environment. He has a long history of substance abuse, primarily alcoholism. His friends participate in and enable Lewis's chemical dependence. Although his family is supportive, they are frustrated by his ongoing struggles with alcohol. Lewis and his family demonstrate decreased understanding regarding his current medical status and future abilities. Lewis's home is inaccessible.

Intervention

Intervention Plan

Collaborative Client Goals That Are Objective and Measurable

At this time, Lewis is unable to state any personal goals. Lewis has anticipated duration of treatment at least 3 weeks with an estimated frequency of 1-2 treatment sessions per week. By the time of discharge, Lewis will perform the following:

1. Sit on the edge of the bed with maximum support while keeping his eyes open
2. Maintain full upper-extremity range of motion (ROM) through exercise and positioning
3. Turn his head in response to his name or other personal information 75% of the time

By the time of discharge, Lewis's family will perform the following:

1. Demonstrate a good understanding of ways to increase level of responsiveness and engagement in environment
2. Demonstrate positioning and range of motion programs using handouts for guidance

Discharge Needs and Plan

Lewis is unable at this time to articulate any goals or discharge plan because of his decreased level of arousal and responsiveness. His family wants to take him home, but they are uncertain about what level of support they can provide. Lewis will need to be medically stable, maintain ROM, establish a means of communicating as able, and tolerate a higher level of intensity of rehabilitation to progress toward being discharged to home. It is anticipated that after leaving the acute care hospital setting, he will need ongoing OT.

Intervention Implementation

Therapeutic Use of Occupations and Activities

Occupation-Based Activities

Mobility
    Bed mobility with log rolling
    Side lying to sitting at edge of bed

Leisure
    Respond to American Indian symbols
    Listen to stories of American Indian folklore

Purposeful Activities

Open eyes to stimuli

Turn head to command or stimuli

Sit up for increasing periods of time

Preparatory Methods

Range of motion

Positioning

Minimally responsive stimulation

Consultation Process

Collaborate with sister and her family regarding safe discharge plan to take care of Lewis at home

Education Process

Train sister in range of motion and positioning programs

Train sister in cognitive retraining to increase level of responsiveness

Provide education regarding current level of abilities and plans for upgrading as ability to engage in environment increases

Intervention Review

Daily informal meetings set with OT to review progress, review treatment plan, and make modifications as needed.

Outcomes

Besides reviewing progress toward Lewis's objective goals, therapy will focus on his ability to resume participation in roles as son, brother, friend, and possibly American Indian community center member.

Questions

1. It is your first time treating Lewis. You are concerned about his medical stability and ability to participate in therapy. How would you determine more about what Lewis can and cannot do during your session?

2. You arrive at Lewis's room to find that because of anxiety he is having difficulty weaning off of the vent. The nurse recommends that you return at a different time. Given your background understanding about his case, is there anything you might be able to do or offer that might help to decrease his anxiety and allow him to wean more successfully?

3. As a new practitioner, you are nervous about Lewis's many monitors and lines. How might you overcome your anxiety during your initial treatment sessions?

4. You find that Lewis is on an air mattress that is not working. What do you do?

5. What are some medical concerns that you might need to be aware of regarding proper positioning for Lewis?

6. You return to find that Lewis is more responsive. What would your plan be to establish a way for him to communicate, knowing that he is unable to vocalize audibly due to the vent?

7. A part of working in an acute care hospital setting is being creative and resourceful. What items might you find in Lewis's hospital room that could be incorporated into a treatment session focused on building strength and endurance? How might you make the exercises motivating to Lewis?

8. What negative adjustment issues might you observe in Lewis the longer he stays in the ICU? How might you help Lewis and his family guard against these issues?

George

ACUTE CARE

Level of Difficulty: Difficult

Overview: Requires understanding of treatment of an adult with a dual diagnosis of spinal cord injury and brain injury with limited support system in an acute care setting

---

Engagement in Occupation to Support Participation in Context(s)

Performance in Areas of Occupation: Full-time employee, adult son, father, and boyfriend

Primary Impairments and Functional Deficits: Decreased medical stability, strength, coordination, mobility, sensation, energy, cognition, understanding of the effect of spinal cord and brain injuries

Context: Divorced adult Caucasian man with a serious girlfriend

Occupational Profile

George is a 47-year-old right-handed man who sustained both spinal cord and moderate brain injuries during a motorcycle crash. He was not helmeted and lost consciousness for at least 5 minutes. He entered the trauma center with a Glasgow Coma Scale (GCS) of 11. His blood levels did not demonstrate signs of alcohol or other substances. His trauma resulted in C5-6 level AIS (ASIA Impairment Scale) A tetraplegia and moderate brain injury. Initially his cervical spine was surgically stabilized with a posterior and anterior approach for a cervical fusion. He received conservative management after the stabilization by having a halo vest placed, which he will need to wear for at least 3 months. He also had a tracheostomy placed due to respiratory complications from the injury. George has a right chest tube drain and a Foley catheter. At night, he needs to be on oxygen with humidity to enable effective breathing through his tracheostomy.

His acute care course has been complicated by a pulmonary embolism (PE) and pneumonia. As a result, he has been treated aggressively with Heparin and respiratory therapies.

George lives alone in a multiple-level home. He works full-time in a biochemistry lab as a technician. George is divorced and has partial custody of his son, Matthew, who stays with him on the weekends. George and his ex-spouse get along fairly well, especially regarding the joint parenting of their son. George has been involved in a

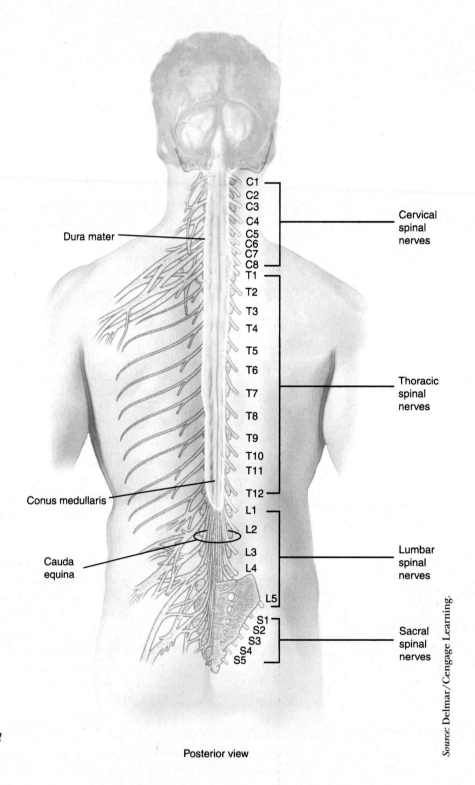

C1
C2
C3
C4
C5
C6
C7
C8

} Cervical
spinal
nerves

Dura mater

T1
T2
T3
T4
T5
T6
T7
T8
T9
T10
T11
T12

} Thoracic
spinal
nerves

Conus medullaris

L1
L2
L3
L4
L5

} Lumbar
spinal
nerves

Cauda
equina

S1
S2
S3
S4
S5

} Sacral
spinal
nerves

Posterior view

Source: Delmar/Cengage Learning.

*The spinal nerves of the central
nervous system.*

serious relationship with Mary for the past 3 years. When George is not working, he
enjoys golfing, gardening, and riding motorcycles.

George is not completely medically stable, therefore he needs to remain in
the acute care hospital setting until it is determined that he is a candidate for a
skilled nursing facility (SNF), inpatient rehabilitation, or home health care (HHC).

George was found to be an ideal candidate for evaluation and treatment by acute care OT, PT, psychology, and SLP. George was also assessed by the acute care OT and PT team and found to be an excellent candidate for further rehabilitation. He is dependent for all of his care and has cognitive issues because of his brain injury. He is to be seen by OT, PT, therapeutic recreation specialists, case management, nursing, physiatry, and psychology services for acute management of his brain and spinal cord injuries.

Analysis of Occupational Performance

Synthesis of Occupational Profile

George is a 47-year-old right-handed man in a halo vest with complete C5-6 level AIS A tetraplegia and moderate brain injury. He lives alone, although he has a significant other who is supportive and interested in providing assistance, if necessary, upon hospital discharge. He works full-time in a biochemistry lab as a technician. He is divorced, but he remains deeply involved with his son and has an amicable relationship with his ex-wife. George's parents are older and live out of state; however, they are emotionally supportive. OT will treat him with a frequency of 2x/week in the acute care setting to address improved communication and participation in his environment while preventing potential secondary complications of brain and spinal cord injuries. George, his significant other, and family members present with an overall decreased understanding regarding his spinal cord and brain injuries and their effects on his current and future function.

Activities of Daily Living

Bathing: George is dependent for his bathing activities. Because of cognitive issues, George has difficulty following instructions from caregivers, and he can be combative at times. He requires maximum cues (both verbal and physical) to stay on task when directed. Additionally, he is not yet able to direct his own care at all.

Bowel and Bladder Management: Graded on the American Spinal Injury Association Impairment Scale (AIS) as C5-6 AIS A (motor and sensory complete at level of injury), George is unable to control his bowels or bladder. George is currently incontinent and has a bowel movement frequently throughout the day and night with no apparent pattern to the accidents. He has not been started on a bowel program. He is at risk of developing an ileus if his bowels are not managed medically and physically for him at this time. He currently has a Foley catheter that he is unable to manage. The Foley will most likely remain inserted until he is discharged to another setting.

Dressing: He is dependent for his dressing tasks. George stays in a hospital gown and adult incontinence briefs all day and night. He does not know how to instruct his caregivers in the steps of how to get him dressed. When he is rolled side to side or the head of the hospital bed is elevated, George complains of dizziness.

Eating/Feeding: He is dependent for all eating tasks. George is at risk for aspiration, and he has already had issues with pneumonia during his short stay in acute care. He is being followed closely by speech language pathology regarding concerns about his dysphagia. He is receiving nutrition from intravenous fluids. He is also being fed a modified diet of pureed solids and honey-thick liquids.

Grooming: For grooming, he is dependent. George cannot hold onto a toothbrush, comb, shaver, or washcloth at this point to perform his grooming. He has difficulty with dizziness when sitting upright and is also at risk for pressure sores, so the nursing assistants or his family perform his grooming for him from bed level.

Functional Mobility: George is dependent for his mobility. Other than getting up for medical procedures and tests, George has not been able to get up out of bed. He becomes dizzy when the head of the hospital bed is elevated more than 30 degrees. When going to procedures, George is transferred from his bed to the hospital gurney, being moved while in a supine position by a transfer slip sheet and the help of three people.

Sexual Activity: George was sexually active and seriously involved with his girlfriend, Mary. Currently, he is unable to engage in sexual activity because of his injury, precautions, and decreased comprehension. He cannot feel anything below his level of injury. He is unaware if he will be able to achieve an erection, let alone ejaculate at this time.

Sleep/Rest: Since his injury, George has had difficulty getting a full night's sleep because of confusion and interruptions. He is on a bed that rotates him from side to side to prevent development of pressure sores or other secondary medical complications. Because he does not sleep well at night, George can be more confused and tends to sleep a lot during the day.

Toilet Hygiene: George is dependent for all toileting tasks. He is unable to manage his clothes or wipe himself. He is currently incontinent and has bowel movements several times throughout the day and night. He has not been started on a bowel program. He also has a Foley catheter and is unable to manage care around his Foley.

Instrumental Activities of Daily Living

Community Mobility: Before his injury, George drove; but because of his current physical and cognitive deficits he depends on others for his community mobility. Although public transportation is accessible in his area, he is unfamiliar with how to access it. Furthermore, George has not yet been able to get up into a wheelchair for basic mobility.

Health Management and Maintenance: George is having difficulties understanding anything about the medications that he is being given, including medications that he took and was familiar with before his crash. He is unable to hold his medications in his hand and he cannot recall what he is taking or when to take it. Before his injury, George went to his doctor annually and made sure to keep his hypertension and diabetes under control.

Home Establishment and Management: George is dependent for home tasks currently. George was responsible for all home management before his injury. He especially enjoyed taking care of his lawn and garden.

Meal Preparation and Cleanup: George was able to make simple, hot meals for himself and his girlfriend Mary. Meal preparation and cleanup is not a core occupation area at this time while he is in the acute care setting.

Education

Formal Educational Participation: George graduated from college with a major in biology.

Work

Employment Interests and Pursuits: Before his injury, George was working full-time as a research technician in a biochemistry lab. His work demands involve frequent use of fine motor control; light lifting, and high-level communication.

Leisure

Leisure Exploration: George is uncertain of leisure options that are available to people who have had a spinal cord and brain injuries. He does not know where to begin to ask questions about leisure options that are available to him.

Leisure Participation: George enjoys gardening, golfing, and riding motorcycles. He is currently uncertain what parts of his leisure he can participate in or what other novel options are available to him.

Social Participation

Family: George's parents are still living, but they live in a different town. They are older and, although emotionally supportive, they cannot provide support to George upon discharge. George still remains in contact with his ex-wife, especially regarding decisions about their son Matthew. George shares custody of Matthew, and before his crash they would spend weekends together. George has been involved with Mary for the past 3 years. She is extremely supportive of him and is hoping to be able to help to take care of George after discharge.

Peer, Friend: George has many friends, but they are nervous about coming to the hospital because they are not sure of his medical stability. They are also having difficulties seeing George so confused.

Factors Influencing Performance Skills and Patterns

Motor Skills

Posture: George's balance is poor in that he is dependent on other people or equipment to keep him from falling over. He is unable to tolerate sitting up in bed with the head of the bed elevated beyond 30 degrees. He has not been able to get into a wheelchair yet because of this inability to tolerate upright/sitting (i.e., sitting at 90 degrees) for prolonged periods of time. He gets dizzy quickly if sitting up past 30 degrees. His postural control is limited further by his halo vest.

Mobility: As stated previously, George's complete spinal cord injury leaves him unable to stand or walk. He will need to work toward building up his ability to being upright and get into an appropriate wheelchair to progress his mobility.

Coordination: George is right-handed. Because of his injury, he has poor gross motor coordination and severely decreased fine motor coordination. He has trace wrist extensors and is not a candidate for learning tenodesis function at this point.

Strength and Effort: George's muscle strength is as follows: shoulder flexion: 4-/5, shoulder abduction: 3/5, shoulder extension: 4/5, elbow flexion: 4-/5, elbow extension: 0/5, supination: 2/5, pronation: 0/5, wrist flexion: 0/5, wrist extension: 1/5, finger flexion: 0/5, finger extension: 0/5. George does not have any movement below his level of injury.

Energy: George has extremely poor endurance. He gets fatigued trying to breathe, especially when secretions become loose and he has to try to cough them up. He needs frequent rest breaks throughout a 30-minute therapy session.

Process Skills

As a result of losing consciousness at the time of his injury, George is demonstrating impairments in several areas of cognitive function. He is having difficulty with attention (select, alternating, and divided), memory, organization, sequencing, functional problem solving, and error identification.

Communication/Interaction Skills

George is able to communicate his basic needs and discuss complex issues most of the time. He does have difficulty following conversations and communicating his thoughts if there are distractions (e.g., visual, auditory). He is unable to write or type at this time due to decreased fine motor control and lack of exposure to adaptive writing equipment.

Habits and Routines

George has had complete disruption of his habits and routines. Not only does his physical condition make it challenging to engage in habits and routines, but also his decreased cognition makes it difficult to recall what used to be automatic.

Roles

Because of the changes in his physical and cognitive abilities, George is having difficulties in his roles as son, father, worker, and boyfriend. He is uncertain what he will do without the use of his hands, and how he will be able to stand, walk, or have sex.

Factors Influencing Context(s)

Cultural

George is Caucasian. He values his family, especially his son. George also prides himself in his ability to work.

Physical

George lives alone in an inaccessible home with many physical barriers to his current abilities.

Social

George's parents are still living, but they are not able to provide much physical assistance owing to their own health conditions and age. George is divorced, but he stays in contact with his ex-wife and their son. George's girlfriend Mary is committed to supporting George throughout his rehabilitation process.

Personal

George is a 47-year-old working right-handed man involved in a committed relationship.

Synthesis of Abilities and Deficits

Facilitators to Occupational Performance

George appears motivated to get stronger and learn how to do things for himself again. He has an emotionally supportive social network, especially his parents and girlfriend. George has had some return of motor function into his upper extremities and is showing trace signs of use of his wrists, which may allow him to manipulate items in his environment better. George's girlfriend is currently committed to learning how to provide physical assistance and hopes to be able to help care for him at discharge.

Barriers to Occupational Performance

Although George's family is supportive, they have limited ability to help with physical assistance or to provide 24-hour supervision if needed. George's cognitive dysfunction may prove to make new learning more challenging. At this point in time, his spinal cord injury is complete and he is physically unable to do any parts of his daily occupations.

Intervention

Intervention Plan

Collaborative Client Goals That Are Objective and Measurable

George is unable to articulate his goals for acute care therapy. He is frustrated that he cannot understand people well and communicate with them. He is also frustrated at not being able to do anything for himself.

George has an anticipated duration of treatment at least 1-2 weeks with an anticipated frequency of 2 treatment sessions per week. By the time of discharge, George will perform the following:

1. Be able to call the nurse for assistance using a sip and puff call light
2. Communicate with parents and friends using a speakerphone with minimal cues
3. Sit up in an appropriate manual wheelchair for at least 30 minutes at a time with decreased report of dizziness and stable vital signs
4. Be able to verbally direct others in his cares (e.g., dressing, grooming, bathing) with moderate to maximal verbal cues
5. Verbalize basic understanding of spinal cord injury education (e.g., pressure relief, orthostatic hypotension, neuroanatomy related to injury level)

By the time of discharge, George's girlfriend will perform the following:

1. Demonstrate good understanding of George's need for range of motion and positioning in bed and in a wheelchair

Discharge Needs and Plan

George's confusion leads to his uncertainty of his future plans and discharge needs. Mary is interested in learning how to care for George. Unfortunately, George's house is inaccessible, so they will have to discuss plans for remodeling the home or come up with a temporary plan. Both George and Mary will need to go through extensive training regarding spinal cord and brain injuries. It is likely that George will need to go to either inpatient rehabilitation or a skilled nursing facility for additional rehabilitation. Regardless of the final discharge plan, George will continue to receive ongoing OT services.

Intervention Implementation

Therapeutic Use of Occupations and Activities

Occupation-Based Activities

Verbal direction of skin inspection, grooming, feeding, dressing, bathing

Pressure relief

Facilitation of mobility

Purposeful Activities

Adaptive phone and call light access

Verbal direction of functional transfers

Preparatory Methods

Biofeedback and neuromuscular electrical stimulation (NMES) to both arms, especially both wrists

Orthotics and splinting for both hands

Fine and gross motor coordination

Stretching and strengthening programs

Positioning programs

Cognitive retraining

Consultation Process

Collaborate to determine the following:

　Safest discharge setting

　Best equipment for accessing nursing staff

　Best equipment for increasing communication with family and friends

Education Process

Family training about assistance and supervision needs

Education about spinal cord injury (bowel, bladder, skin, pressure relief, neuroanatomy of injury level, orthostatic hypotension, autonomic dysreflexia, and sexual function)

Education about brain injury (neuroanatomy and physiology, behavioral management, cognitive effects, influence of medications)

Initial nutrition counseling, especially related to bowel management and healthy healing after spinal cord and brain injury

Intervention Review

Daily informal meetings set with OT to review progress, review treatment plan, and make modifications as needed.

Outcomes

Along with reviewing progress toward George's objective goals, therapy will focus on his ability to resume participation in his roles of father, son, and boyfriend.

Questions

1. You enter George's hospital room and notice that he is having difficulty breathing, cannot talk, and is turning blue. You suspect that he is throwing a mucus plug; what do you do?

2. The primary nurse and emergency response team enter to deal with George's decreased responsiveness. What is your responsibility in this situation?

3. What are the steps that you would take to help build up George's upright tolerance so he can get out of bed and participate in more aspects of therapy and ultimately engage with his environment better?

4. Create a "Get Up and Go Schedule" for George, his family, and the nursing staff so that he is slowly able to overcome orthostatic hypotension and get up into his wheelchair 2-3 times per day.

5. You notice that George is complaining of getting anxious about having further complications with breathing. What could you incorporate into your therapy sessions to help with breathing and George's emotional health?

6. Along with providing training in environmental controls of the call light and phone, what else might you incorporate into George's therapy program so that he can access his environment better?

7. What are some considerations you might have regarding moving George around with the numerous lines that he has attached to him?

8. What are some medical concerns specific to George's brain and spinal cord injuries that you will need to be aware of while providing care and education?

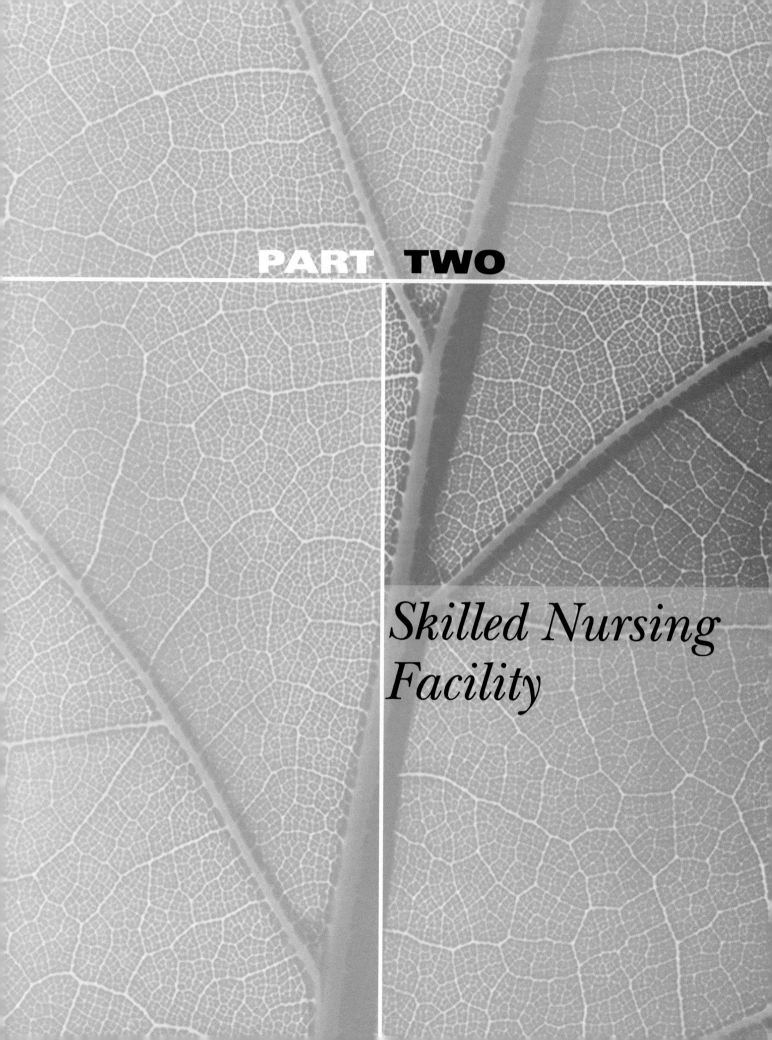

PART TWO

Skilled Nursing Facility

CASE STUDY 5

Carolina

SKILLED NURSING FACILITY

Level of Difficulty: Easy

Overview: Requires understanding of precautions related to knee replacement including teaching use of adaptive equipment to a woman after total knee replacement in a skilled nursing facility setting

---

Engagement in Occupation to Support Participation in Context(s)

Performance in Areas of Occupation: Spouse, mother, grandmother, retiree, amateur tennis player, and church member

Primary Impairments and Functional Deficits: Pain, generalized weakness, decreased flexion and extension of knee, decreased ability to manage stairs, decreased understanding of how to incorporate knee precautions into daily activities

Context: Married retired 65-year-old Spanish-speaking woman

Occupational Profile

Carolina is a 65-year-old married Spanish-speaking woman who has severe degenerative arthritis in her left knee. She has been less able to engage in daily exercise, and now the pain in her knee is limiting her ability to perform parts of her daily occupations such as standing for periods of time in church, kneeling to wash the floor, or running to play amateur tennis. She was found to be a candidate for a total knee arthroplasty. The surgery was uncomplicated; she stayed briefly in acute care for a few days to monitor her medical stability.

Carolina lives with her spouse in a split-level home with many stairs. She is not able to stay on the main level because there is no bedroom or bathroom and she does not want to sleep on a pull-out couch. In order to take a shower, she would have to be able to manage stairs; she has access to both a walk-in shower on the lower level and a tub/shower combination on the upper level. She loves to take baths, but has been told that she will be unable to soak her knee for at least one month after the surgery. She is the primary cook and takes care of the home management tasks except for lawn care and taking out the trash, which her spouse does.

Carolina used to work in a factory in an assembly line, but she has just retired. She is Catholic, is active in her local church, and attends mass regularly. Many of

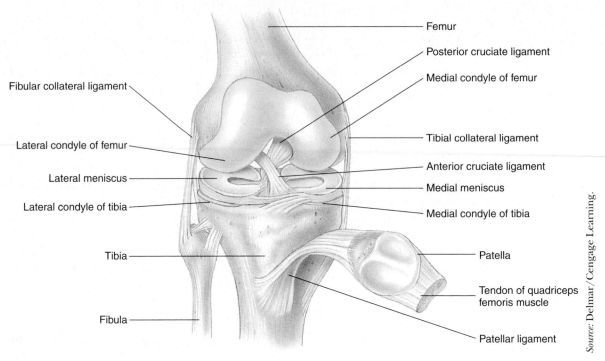

Femur
Posterior cruciate ligament
Medial condyle of femur
Tibial collateral ligament
Anterior cruciate ligament
Medial meniscus
Medial condyle of tibia
Patella
Tendon of quadriceps femoris muscle
Patellar ligament

Fibular collateral ligament
Lateral condyle of femur
Lateral meniscus
Lateral condyle of tibia
Tibia
Fibula

Source: Delmar/Cengage Learning.

Anterior view of the knee joint.

her friends in the area are from her church. Throughout the mass, Carolina needs to stand for prolonged periods of time and genuflect several times. As her pain and endurance became worse, Carolina was less able to stand or genuflect, and close to the time of the surgery she became reluctant to attend masses.

Carolina and her spouse have two grown children; one lives nearby but works full-time and the other lives out of state. Her eldest child, a daughter, has two children, for whom Carolina provides day care 3 days a week.

Carolina had been active playing tennis and upon retiring pursued amateur status. When she was feeling better, she would play doubles tennis at least 3 times per week. As the pain increased, she was less able to play tennis and finally had to stop playing. This contributed to Carolina becoming generally weakened. She would love to have success with her knee replacement and return to playing amateur tennis at least one to two times per week.

According to the acute care notes, Carolina is functioning at a reasonable level except for needing additional time to work on lower body dressing, bathing, stairs, and identifying equipment needs for discharge to home. Furthermore, Carolina's spouse has received initial training, but he would benefit from additional reinforcement in case he needs to help her at home with any specific care.

Since Carolina has determined that she cannot go directly home from acute care, she is transitioning for a short stay at a skilled nursing facility closer to her home. Carolina is now medically stable and has been evaluated by acute occupational and physical therapy and found to be an excellent candidate for a short 3- to 5-day stay at the skilled nursing facility for ongoing OT twice a day. She is being admitted to the facility to be seen by OT, PT, CM, nursing, and physiatry.

Analysis of Occupational Performance

Synthesis of Occupational Profile

Carolina is a 65-year-old married Spanish-speaking woman status post left total knee replacement. She is a retiree, spouse, mother, grandmother, church member, and amateur tennis player. She presents for OT at the skilled nursing facility to address equipment needs and use for resuming participation in the following areas of occupation: lower body dressing, bathing, meal preparation, and stair management.

Observed Performance in Desired Occupation/Activity

Activities of Daily Living

Bathing: Carolina requires moderate assistance; she is able to wash her upper body, but she needs help to wash her left lower leg, foot, and bottom. Because of pain and decreased energy, she sits on a shower chair for the majority of the time.

Dressing: She is independent with upper body dressing but needs moderate assistance with lower body dressing; she is able to get her underwear and pants onto her right leg, but she needs assistance to get them over her right leg. She can stand up with minimal assistance and pull her pants up the rest of the way. She cannot put on her socks or shoes without assistance because of decreased tolerance and range to bend her left knee.

Functional Mobility: Carolina needs minimal assistance for stand pivot transfer to get up into standing. Carolina is then able to walk about 50 feet with a rolling walker with stand-by assistance.

Toileting: She needs minimal assistance; she is able to manage her clothing before going to the bathroom, but she needs to hold onto the toilet safety frame. She is able to wipe herself thoroughly with the assistance of a raised toilet seat and toilet safety frame. Carolina requires assistance to get up into standing and then is able to pull her clothing up after using the toilet.

Instrumental Activities of Daily Living

Community Mobility: Currently, Carolina is not able to walk outside because of decreased energy, pain, and fear of her knee giving out. The terrain around her home is fairly level. Before her knee surgery, she drove a car.

Health Management and Maintenance: Carolina needs additional training with managing her medications because of the language barrier and difficulty having her medication instructions listed in Spanish. While at the skilled nursing facility, Carolina would like to be able to learn to perform self-medication.

Home Establishment and Management; Meal Preparation and Cleanup: Carolina performs the cooking and cleanup at home. Carolina has not been able to tolerate sessions in the kitchen because of pain, decreased endurance, and nausea in the presence of food.

Education

Formal Educational Participation: Carolina did not complete high school; she met her future spouse, got married, and started a family.

Work

Job Performance: Carolina worked in a factory on the assembly line. She retired when she was 62 years old.

Retirement Adjustment: Carolina had been adjusting well to retirement and had been active playing amateur tennis and taking care of her grandchildren three times per week. As her pain increased, she was less able to engage in these activities, which has made being retired more of a challenge.

Leisure

Leisure Participation: As stated before, Carolina has been actively involved in amateur doubles tennis and played at least three times per week until her pain became too much to bear. Carolina also enjoys sewing, socializing with friends, and watching movies.

Social Participation

Community: Carolina is strongly connected to her Catholic faith. She is closely involved with her church community and is an active member, except for recently attending mass less often because of pain.

Family: Carolina has been married for 47 years. She and her spouse have a good relationship. Carolina's children are grown and have their own families. Her daughter's family lives in town while her son and his spouse live out of state. Carolina provides day care for her daughter's children three times per week. This was becoming more challenging because of pain, decreased mobility, and decreased endurance.

Peer, Friend: Carolina's friends are important to her and are mainly from her church community or tennis club. When her friends found out that she was having surgery, they offered to help by bringing meals.

Factors Influencing Performance Skills and Patterns

Motor Skills

Mobility: Carolina's mobility is decreased by pain and generalized weakness. She is able to walk around only with a rolling walker at this time. She is able to get up and down from various surfaces, but she needs minimal assistance. Carolina and her spouse want to determine the best equipment to buy for bathing/showering. She is unable to manage stairs or step into a walk-in shower. Carolina is lacking range in both flexion and extension of her left knee.

Strength and Effort: After the knee surgery, Carolina demonstrates slightly decreased strength in her left leg especially at her hip flexor, knee flexor, and knee extensor.

Energy: Carolina was less able to move around because of pain and generalized weakness before her surgery. As a result of this and the actual surgery, her energy is fair for her daily activities. She has had difficulty with nausea and vomiting, which are further affecting her energy and ability to engage in her daily occupations.

Process Skills

Knowledge: Carolina is able to state her knee precautions, but she is not able to incorporate them consistently into such tasks as lower body dressing or bathing. She does not speak nor understand much English, therefore an interpreter is necessary for all training and education.

Habits and Routines

Because of her knee precautions and lack of knee range, Carolina's morning and evening routines related to lower body dressing and bathing have been disrupted.

Roles

Carolina is unable to engage completely in her roles as grandmother, as day care provider, as church member, or as amateur tennis player until she has community mobility and can stand for prolonged periods of time.

Factors Influencing Context(s)

Cultural

Carolina has a strong Catholic faith system.

Physical

At home, to get to her shower or bedroom, Carolina needs to manage a flight of stairs using one railing. She needs to be able to stand and genuflect to be able to participate fully during Catholic masses.

Social

Her spouse is supportive although he is unfamiliar with performing such tasks as cooking or cleaning. Carolina's church members and friends from the tennis club are already asking what things they could do to help her as she recovers at home, including providing meals.

Personal

Carolina is a 65-year-old married, retired Spanish-speaking woman.

Synthesis of Abilities and Deficits

Facilitators to Occupational Performance

Carolina is able to verbalize her knee precautions. The knee surgery was uncomplicated and she is healing quickly. Carolina has a supportive spouse. Carolina is able to walk short distances using a rolling walker. Before her pain got to be too great, Carolina had kept active playing tennis and taking care of her grandchildren.

Barriers to Occupational Performance

Carolina is experiencing pain, decreased knee range of motion, and was generally weakened before her surgery. To shower or get to her bedroom, she needs to be able to manage several stairs, and so far she has been unable to manage stairs. Although she demonstrates ability to state her knee precautions, Carolina has yet to learn how to use equipment to incorporate the precautions into lower dressing and bathing.

Intervention

Intervention Plan

Collaborative Client Goals That Are Objective and Measurable

Carolina has an anticipated duration of treatment 4-6 days, with an estimated frequency of 3-5 treatment sessions. By the time of discharge, Carolina will perform the following:

1. Lower body dressing with modified independence and adaptive equipment
2. Toileting with independence
3. Functional transfers (bed, toilet, shower, car) with independence from an ambulatory level with appropriate assistive device and durable medical equipment
4. Bathing with independence and appropriate adaptive and durable medical equipment
5. Good understanding of knee precautions during daily routine including hot meal preparation

By the time of discharge, Carolina's family will perform the following:

1. Demonstrate good understanding of equipment needs for discharge

Discharge Needs and Plan

Carolina is planning to return home. She needs to be able to learn how to use adaptive equipment to incorporate knee precautions. She needs to be able to manage stairs. She will need to buy adaptive and durable medical equipment before discharge. Carolina's spouse is available to help on a limited basis if needed and will benefit from additional education and training. It is anticipated that after leaving the skilled nursing facility, she will not need any further OT.

Intervention Implementation

Therapeutic Use of Occupations and Activities

Occupation-Based Activities

Lower body dressing

Bathing/showering

Toileting

Functional transfers (car, bed, shower, toilet)

Meal preparation and cleanup

Light home management

Health management and maintenance

Purposeful Activities

Practice putting on socks and shoes

Practice putting on underwear and pants with reacher and progress to no reacher

Practice unmaking and making a bed

Practice frying an egg while standing

Practice stepping into and out of a walk-in shower

Preparatory Methods

Physical agent modalities: ice

Continuous passive range of motion machine

Exercise: Calisthenics while standing and activities that promote flexion and extension of knee

Consultation Process

Collaborating to determine safest equipment needs for lower body dressing and bathing

Education Process

Client and family training of equipment recommendations

Education of knee precautions during daily activities

Education regarding home modifications for occupations such as cooking

Intervention Review

Daily informal meetings set with OT to review progress, review treatment plan, and make modifications as needed.

Outcomes

Besides reviewing progress toward Carolina's objective goals, therapy will focus on her ability to resume participation in her roles as spouse, grandmother, amateur tennis player, and church member.

Questions

1. Carolina is getting ready to return home. What would be an additional area necessary to address especially if her knee replacement had been to her right knee instead of her left knee?

2. List some different functional activities that you could do with Carolina to encourage flexion and extension of her left knee to complement work done in physical therapy sessions.

3. Because the medical doctor performs rounds only weekly, you get in the habit of checking the International Normalization Ratio (INR) levels, an indicator on the clotting time of blood in response to medications like Coumadin, especially on your orthopedic clients. You note that Carolina's levels are too low (i.e., below 2). What does this put her at risk for and what will you do with this knowledge?

4. If instead, you noted that her levels were too high (i.e., greater than 3), what would this put her at risk for and would you change what you would do? Why or why not?

5. When working on showering with Carolina, you note that her left leg has increased in size, is hot to touch compared to her right leg, and with the knee flexed and passive dorsiflexion, Carolina experiences intense calf pain. What should you suspect? What are your next steps?

6. You feel that when interacting with Carolina and her interpreter that the interpreter is not translating all information and is changing what you and Carolina are saying. What do you do?

References

INR@Home. A New Standard of Care for People on Blood Thinners. (2005). About INR Levels: The Importance of "Staying in Range" to Avoid Serious Complications, at http://www.inrselftest.com/index.php?src=gendocs&link=AboutINRLevels&category=Main.

Urbano, Frank L. (2001). Review of Clinical Signs: Homan's Sign in the Diagnosis of Deep Venous Thrombosis. Hospital Physician, pp. 23- 24, at http://www.turner-white.com/pdf/hp_mar01_homan.pdf. Turner White Communications, Inc. Wayne, PA.

Clarence

SKILLED NURSING FACILITY

Level of Difficulty: Moderate

Overview: Requires understanding of treatment of an elderly person after coronary artery bypass graft (CABG) who is primary caregiver to his spouse with Alzheimer's disease in a skilled nursing facility setting with an uncertain final discharge disposition

Engagement in Occupation to Support Participation in Context(s)

Performance in Areas of Occupation: Spouse and primary caregiver, father, grandfather, church member, and church choir member

Primary Impairments and Functional Deficits: Generalized weakness, decreased understanding regarding sternal precautions, decreased ability to be primary caregiver to spouse with Alzheimer's disease

Context: Elderly married Caucasian man who is primary caregiver of spouse with Alzheimer's disease

Occupational Profile

Clarence is an 85-year-old married man status post triple CABG. Initially, Clarence experienced chest pain with pain radiating down into his left arm. He was admitted to the emergency room and found to have a myocardial infarction as a result of three blocked coronary arteries. It was determined that he would undergo emergency CABG. He tolerated the surgery with minimal complications other than post-operative hypotension.

Clarence has been married for almost 65 years to his spouse, Adelaide. They have four grown sons, two of whom live in the nearby area. The sons and their families have been helping out with heavier chores around the house, grocery shopping, finances, and preparing microwaveable meals. Clarence's spouse has Alzheimer's disease and he has been her primary caregiver for the past 15 years.

Clarence and Adelaide live in an apartment in the independent living center of a senior building. They have a tub/shower combination, small kitchen with a gas oven and stove, two bedrooms, and a living room. The bathroom is accessible with grab bars by the toilet and tub/shower.

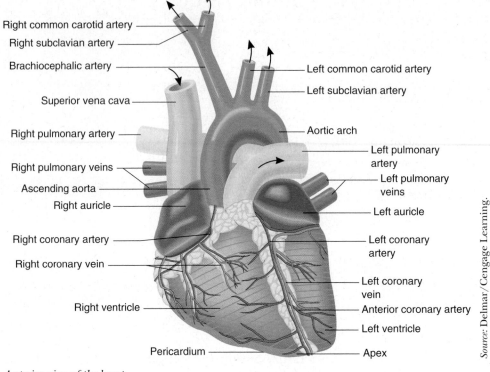

Right common carotid artery
Right subclavian artery
Brachiocephalic artery
Superior vena cava
Right pulmonary artery
Right pulmonary veins
Ascending aorta
Right auricle
Right coronary artery
Right coronary vein
Right ventricle
Pericardium

Left common carotid artery
Left subclavian artery
Aortic arch
Left pulmonary artery
Left pulmonary veins
Left auricle
Left coronary artery
Left coronary vein
Anterior coronary artery
Left ventricle
Apex

Source: Delmar/Cengage Learning.

Anterior view of the heart.

Every week, Clarence and his spouse still attend church, where Clarence sings in the choir. Clarence drives both to church and to various areas around town. He just renewed his license and successfully passed a defensive driving course.

Clarence was in the acute care setting for 5 days and participated in occupational and physical therapy services. Although he improved in his overall function to supervision for functional transfers to and from elevated surfaces, lower body dressing and toileting, and minimum assistance for bathing, he was not functioning independently and safely enough to return home, where he would still have to be the primary caregiver for Adelaide. The acute care team, including Clarence and his children, felt that transitioning temporarily to a SNF would be necessary.

Clarence is transitioning to a SNF with focus on increased independence, safety, and determination of whether he will be able to return to the independent living portion of his senior building or should pursue transitioning to the assisted living facility (ALF) portion of that building. The doctor from the acute care setting has ordered evaluation and treatment for ongoing OT and PT services at the SNF. While at the new facility, Clarence will also receive services from a social worker as well. A doctor will monitor Clarence medically during weekly rounds. If indicated, a psychologist for adjustment to his current medical condition and ongoing issues with caregiving for Adelaide may also see Clarence on a weekly basis.

Analysis of Occupational Performance

Synthesis of Occupational Profile

Clarence is an 85-year-old married man who sustained a myocardial infarction and underwent a subsequent CABG x3 secondary to blockage of the coronary arteries. He is the primary caregiver for his spouse, who has Alzheimer's disease. In addition to his primary role as spouse/caregiver, Clarence is also a father, grandfather, and active member of his church. He presents for OT in the SNF to address difficulty with sit to stand transfers, washing, performing home management, overall weakness, and understanding of sternal precautions. The ultimate goal is to upgrade his overall functional skills to independent with an ability to resume caregiving for Adelaide. Furthermore, this temporary placement will be focused on determining Clarence's ability to return to the independent living center at his senior building or whether pursuit of transitioning to the assisted living portion of the senior building would be better suited for Clarence and his spouse.

Observed Performance in Desired Occupation/Activity

Activities of Daily Living

Bathing: He requires minimum assistance to complete bathing tasks. Clarence is able to wash all parts of his body, but he needs help to come into standing from a shower chair as well as to wash and dry his feet. He is able to adhere to his sternal precautions at least 75% of the time, but because of ongoing generalized weakness he uses his arms too much (i.e., more than sternal precautions recommend) when coming to stand. He needs to sit on a chair part of the way through the shower after feeling fatigued. For the rest of time he maintains hold of a grab bar while washing. He is moderately fatigued at the end of the shower.

Bowel and Bladder Management: To avoid straining, Clarence is on Colace, a stool softener. He is no longer having issues of retention and is able to urinate with the help of bladder medication to improve flow. The nurses no longer have to perform straight catheterization.

Dressing: Clarence can be characterized as independent with increased time for upper body dressing tasks. Clarence is able to stand up and walk to obtain his clothes as long as his bed his high enough for him to stand without assistance. Clarence currently needs supervision for lower body dressing. He is able to get his underwear and pants started and pull them up over his hips and bottom with a noticeable need for increased time (i.e., over 30 minutes). He is unable to put on his compression hose independently, but he can now put on and take off his shoes within 3 to 5 minutes.

Functional Mobility: For overall functional mobility, the amount of assistance Clarence requires varies from minimum assistance to supervision. He is able to roll to both sides when in bed and maintain his sternal precautions and no longer needs help other than a bed rail to get from his side up into sitting. Clarence is better able to stand up from sitting when the surface is elevated. However, due to ongoing generalized weakness, he continues to have difficulty standing up from sitting on standard height or lower surfaces (i.e., 21 inches or lower). Clarence remembers his sternal precautions 75% of the time, but he is weak and needs to use his arms to stand up from low surfaces. After getting up, he is able to walk 100-150' without any assistive device (AD), with supervision.

Sexual Activity: In spite of Adelaide's dementia, Clarence and his spouse have kept a relatively active level of intimacy. Clarence continues to be concerned how his heart surgery will affect their intimacy and whether he should be worried about another myocardial infarction when they are having sex.

Sleep/Rest: Although Clarence was initially sleeping better in the hospital because he did not have to be concerned about Adelaide's wandering, he has now been having more difficulties sleeping because of anxiety about whether they will be able to return home or need to move into an alternative setting such as the assisted living portion of their building for seniors.

Toileting: Clarence requires supervision to carry out his toileting tasks. He is able to get his clothing down before going to the toilet. He no longer needs help to wipe himself after a bowel movement. Clarence needs to be on an elevated toilet seat to stand without assistance and then can get his clothing back up without assistance.

Instrumental Activities of Daily Living

Care of Others: As noted earlier, Clarence has been the primary caregiver for his spouse for the past 15 years. As her dementia has progressed, he has helped her more and has taken over most of the responsibilities around the house. As Clarence has been healing from his bypass, he has become more anxious about whether he will be able to continue to be the primary caregiver for his spouse, especially if they return to their apartment.

Community Mobility: Clarence drove before this hospitalization. He recently successfully passed a defensive driving course when he renewed his license. While he is unable to drive because of his sternal precautions and the demands on the incision and healing bone for the next 4 to 6 weeks, Clarence's sons have stated that they are willing to drive their parents to church and medical appointments including follow-up cardiac rehabilitation as needed.

Financial Management: As care of Adelaide increased, Clarence relinquished control of his finances to his eldest son, a tax accountant.

Health Management and Maintenance: Clarence had been managing his own medications for hypertension, blood thinner, cholesterolemia, and diuretic premorbidly. He went to his doctor for annual physicals. After his bypass surgery, Clarence is on a few different medications and the cardiologist has changed dosages of his previous medications. Clarence is in need of being evaluated regarding his ability to administer his medications independently.

Home Establishment and Management; Meal Preparation and Cleanup: Prior to admit (PTA) Clarence was in charge of all areas regarding home management and meal preparation, although his children would bring microwaveable frozen meals. Currently, Clarence is unable to perform any of this because of decreased endurance. He currently needs to learn how to change his and his spouse's diet to account for cardiac concerns related to lower cholesterol, fat, and sodium intake.

Safety Procedures and Emergency Responses: Clarence is aware of safety and emergency procedures related to his and his spouse's health. Clarence is better able to get around from elevated surfaces, so he is now following his sternal precautions better and more safely. Currently, Clarence needs to work on increasing his ability to follow his sternal precautions with 100% accuracy (at 75% right now). He needs to be able to demonstrate how to take care of Adelaide safely. He needs to be able to move quickly enough without falling to get out of his apartment in case of an emergency.

Shopping: Clarence has help from his sons and their families for the majority of their shopping needs.

Education

Formal Educational Participation: Clarence has a high school education.

Work

Retirement Preparation and Adjustment: Clarence is a retired insurance salesman. Although he saved well for his retirement, Clarence and Adelaide are on a fixed income.

Leisure

Leisure Participation: Clarence enjoys getting together with other people in the building for seniors. Despite his increasing care for Adelaide, he tries to attend the center's various events and activities within walking distance of the apartment. Clarence used to enjoy playing cribbage and bridge, but he has not been playing either game recently because of responsibilities to Adelaide and decreased endurance.

Social Participation

Community: Clarence is very involved in his church as a church elder and choir member. He tries to remain active with others in his senior building as well.

Family: Clarence has a strong commitment to his marriage and providing care for his spouse. His family, particularly the two sons who live nearby, is supportive of both him and his spouse.

Peer, Friend: Clarence spends time as able with friends in the senior building, but less frequently because taking care of Adelaide has consumed more time and effort.

Factors Influencing Performance Skills and Patterns

Motor Skills

Mobility: Clarence's mobility has been improving although he is still challenged by standing up from standard to lower height surfaces. He continues to benefit from elevated surfaces such as a higher bed or a raised toilet seat. Once standing, he is able to walk 100-150 feet with supervision using no assistive device. Clarence has also been starting to get up at night by himself safely to go to the bathroom. In order to walk safely outside in the community, he needs to be able to walk 2.6 feet per second.

Strength and Effort: Clarence is generally weak all over. His overall strength is 4-/5 throughout both his upper and lower extremities except for his quadriceps and gluteus, which are 3/5.

Energy: Clarence fatigues easily with activity, needing frequent rest breaks; the frequency of breaks has decreased compared to the first days after his bypass surgery. His overall endurance has improved to being able to engage in an activity for 10 minutes before needing to take a rest. During 30 minutes of activity, he takes at least 3 rest breaks. He needs to rest for at least 1 minute before resuming. Clarence has been working on cardiorespiratory capacity necessary for singing a 3-minute hymn.

Process Skills

Knowledge: Clarence is knowledgeable about his previous cardiac issues regarding medication management. However, currently he continues to demonstrate decreased understanding of modifications to his medication routine and how to institute and follow a cardiac diet at home.

Habits and Routines

Clarence's daily routine of getting dressed, bathing, toileting, and taking care of his spouse has been disrupted since the surgery. He is, however, starting to get into a similar morning routine, especially with the knowledge of planning for scheduled therapies throughout his day.

Roles

Clarence is a spouse and caregiver, father, grandfather, and active church member. Due to his surgery and sternal precautions, his role as caregiver to Adelaide has been disrupted. Furthermore, to engage in his role as church choir member, Clarence will need to have one of his son's drive him to church until he is able to return to driving without worry of hurting his sternal incision. If he needs to because of decreased endurance, Clarence will be able to remain seated when singing, but typically choir members stand for periods of about 5 minutes at a time.

Factors Influencing Context(s)

Cultural

Clarence is Caucasian. He values his family and his Christian background. He attends church every Sunday, where he sings in the choir.

Physical

Clarence's primary physical barriers are related to difficulty getting up into standing when sitting on standard to lower surfaces while maintaining sternal precautions. It may be necessary for various surfaces at home to be elevated to increase Clarence's adherence to his precautions.

Social

Clarence prides himself in being incredibly social, although he has been more limited since needing to care more intensely for his spouse. His friends in the senior building are very supportive in offering help and checking in to make sure that Clarence and Adelaide are doing well.

Personal

Clarence is an 85-year-old married man who is the primary caregiver for his spouse, Adelaide.

Synthesis of Abilities and Deficits

Facilitators to Occupational Performance

Clarence is cognitively intact. His sons are supportive and have been helping with heavier home management tasks, finances, and running errands. Clarence recently passed a defensive driving test and has a current driving license. Before his myocardial infarction and subsequent surgery, Clarence maintained his health fairly well. Clarence remains active with his church, especially the church choir. Clarence is better able to get around while following his sternal precautions if standing from elevated surfaces. He is able to walk 100-150 feet without an assistive device.

Barriers to Occupational Performance

Clarence is generally weak not only from his myocardial infarction and surgery, but also from a long history of cardiac problems. The surfaces in Clarence and Adelaide's apartment are too low for him to get up safely independently. Although he has tried to manage his health well, he has not understood how to incorporate a cardiac diet into the meals that he prepares for himself and his spouse. Clarence's spouse has late stage Alzheimer's disease and is unable to provide assistance or supervision. Furthermore, Clarence was and remains his spouse's primary caregiver. Clarence is beginning to realize that he may need additional help to maintain care of Adelaide at home.

Intervention

Intervention Plan

Collaborative Client Goals That Are Objective and Measurable

Clarence has an anticipated duration of treatment for the next 2 to 3 months, with an estimated frequency of two 30-minute sessions at least 5 times per week until discharge. By the time of discharge, Clarence will perform the following:

1. Functional transfers (bed, toilet, tub/shower, car) with independence from elevated surfaces as needed using sternal precautions 100% of the time
2. Bathing with modified independence with adaptive equipment as needed
3. Lower body dressing with independence and 100% adherence to sternal precautions
4. Toileting with independence with an elevated toilet seat
5. Good understanding and incorporation of sternal precautions into daily routine 100% of the time
6. Hot meal preparation using microwave with incorporation of cardiac diet with independence and use of a recipe or checklist as needed
7. Demonstrate good understanding of discharge disposition recommendations regarding equipment, safety, cardiac diet, and home program for endurance

Discharge Needs and Plan

Clarence is planning to return home, but he realizes that all of the surfaces in his apartment will need to be higher. He is also beginning to realize that the level of assistance and supervision he had been providing to his spouse is too high for his current medical condition. He is now more open to considering a move to the assisted living portion of their senior building. He would still like to be extremely independent, because Adelaide has Alzheimer's disease. His children can help with running errands and setting up meals, but they cannot provide consistent assistance and supervision. It is anticipated that after leaving the SNF, Clarence will benefit from ongoing outpatient cardiac rehabilitation.

Intervention Implementation

Therapeutic Use of Occupations and Activities

Occupation-Based Activities

Toileting

Dressing

Bathing/showering

Sexual activity

Care of others

Home management

Health management and maintenance
   Medication management

Mobility
   Sit to stand from various surfaces
   Walking
   Stairs

Purposeful Activities

Practice putting on socks with or without equipment while maintaining sternal precautions

Practice putting on underwear and pants with or without equipment while maintaining sternal precautions

Practice unmaking and making a bed

Functional transfers from various surfaces while maintaining sternal precautions

Practice setting up medications for the week and transition to self-medication routine

Make complete hot meal using recipes from cardiac diet cookbook

Preparatory Methods

Cardiac calisthenics

Exercises

Consultation Process

Collaborate to determine the following:
   Equipment needs for safest dressing, toileting, and bathing

Safe bathing options

Best way to organize weekly medication management

Safest discharge disposition to meet needs of being primary caregiver to spouse with Alzheimer's disease

Education Process

Client and family training regarding recommended equipment

Education about sternal precautions during daily activities

Client and family training regarding meal planning and preparation using cardiac diet

Intervention Review

Daily informal meetings set with OT to review progress, review treatment plan, and make modifications as needed.

Outcomes

In addition to reviewing progress toward Clarence's objective goals, therapy will focus on his ability to resume participation in his roles as spouse and primary caregiver, father, and active church member.

Questions

1. Now that Clarence has transitioned to the SNF, are there any different essential questions that would help guide discharge planning for Clarence as compared to when he was in the acute care setting? What would they be?

2. Would the fact that Clarence has cognitive deficits affect his ability to transition with his spouse to an assisted living facility? Why or why not?

3. How would you design your treatment sessions to help provide information and training regarding whether Clarence should transition to an assisted living facility versus return to his apartment in the independent living portion of the senior building?

4. During your sessions, you continue to monitor Clarence's vitals closely. What vitals would cause you to be concerned? Knowing that the doctor has already made weekly rounds, what would you do if his vitals are abnormal and you suspect that Clarence is having increased cardiac issues?

5. As your treatment sessions progress, it appears that Clarence is still not ready to transition to the assisted living portion of the building for seniors because he will need more supervision/assistance than his fixed income can cover. What are your options?

6. As a standard protocol for the SNF, all residents are screened regarding cognitive and emotional function. You complete the mini mental state examination (MMSE) and determine that he is scoring below 23 points, indicative of cognitive dysfunction. You consult with the OT and determine that further testing is necessary using the Cognitive Performance Test (CPT). Because time is limited, you need to focus on the most relevant topics from the seven categories: medications, dress, shop, toast, phone, wash, and travel. What categories would you choose and why?

7. In working with Clarence, you notice that he appears more anxious because of being more distractible and is having difficulties participating fully in therapy. What do you think might be key factors contributing to his anxiety? You know that the psychologist is only available once a week, what do you do?

References

Bares, K. (1998). Neuropsychological Predictors of Functional Level in Alzheimer's Disease. Unpublished doctoral dissertation. University of Minnesota.

Burns T., Mortimer J.A., and Merchak P. (1994). The Cognitive Performance Test: A New Approach to Functional Assessment in Alzheimer's Disease. *The Journal of Geriatric Psychiatry and Neurology, 7.*

Jennings-Pikey M. (2001). A Validation Study of the Cognitive Performance Test. Unpublished doctoral dissertation. Wheaton College, IL.

Perry, J. (1992). *Gait Analysis Normal and Pathological Functions.* SLACK, Inc. Thorofare, NJ.

Perry, J., Garrett, M., Gronley, J.K., and Mulroy, S.J. (1995). Classification of Walking Handicap in the Stroke Population. *Stroke, 26,* 982–989.

George

SKILLED NURSING FACILITY

Level of Difficulty: Difficult

Overview: Requires understanding of treatment of an adult with a dual diagnosis of spinal cord injury and brain injury with limited support system within a skilled nursing facility (SNF) setting

Engagement in Occupation to Support Participation in Context(s)

Performance in Areas of Occupation: Full-time employee, adult son, father, and boyfriend

Primary Impairments and Functional Deficits: Decreased skin integrity, strength, coordination, mobility, sensation, energy, and cognition; autonomic dysreflexia and orthostatic hypotension; and decreased understanding of the effect of brain and spinal cord injuries

Context: Divorced adult Caucasian man with serious girlfriend

Occupational Profile

George is 47-year-old right-handed male who sustained both spinal cord and mild brain injuries during a motorcycle crash. He was not helmeted and lost consciousness for at least 5 minutes. Upon admission to the trauma center, his GCS was 11. His blood levels did not demonstrate signs of alcohol or other chemical substances. His trauma resulted in C5,6 AIS A tetraplegia and moderate brain injury. Initially his cervical spine was surgically stabilized with hardware using both a posterior and anterior approach. He received conservative management after the stabilization by having a halo vest placed, which he will wear for at least 3 months after stabilization. He also had a tracheostomy placed because of respiratory complications from the injury. His acute care course was made more difficult by a pulmonary embolism (PE) and pneumonia. He was treated with Heparin and aggressive respiratory therapy.

George's care was medically managed and stabilized in an acute care setting over the course of a month. While in acute care, George had a right chest tube drain and a Foley catheter. He continues to be on oxygen with humidity in order to breathe effectively through his tracheostomy.

He was stabilized and then, after a month in acute care, transitioned to inpatient rehabilitation for 5 weeks. There the focus of treatment was on prevention

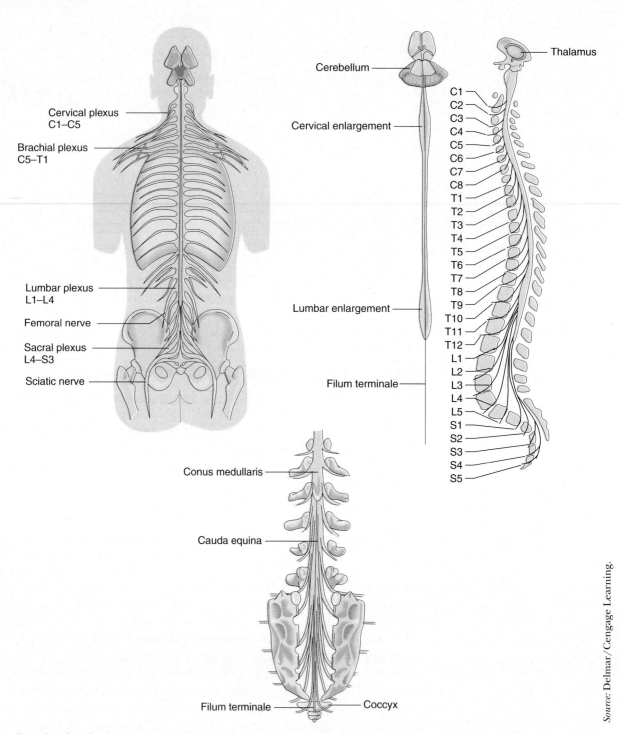

Cerebellum

Thalamus

Cervical plexus
C1–C5

Brachial plexus
C5–T1

Cervical enlargement

C1
C2
C3
C4
C5
C6
C7
C8
T1
T2
T3
T4
T5
T6
T7
T8
T9
T10
T11
T12
L1
L2
L3
L4
L5
S1
S2
S3
S4
S5

Lumbar plexus
L1–L4

Femoral nerve

Lumbar enlargement

Sacral plexus
L4–S3

Sciatic nerve

Filum terminale

Conus medullaris

Cauda equina

Filum terminale

Coccyx

Spinal cord and nerves.

Source: Delmar/Cengage Learning.

of secondary complications of SCI including respiratory management, verbal direction of care, spinal cord and brain injury education, and cognitive retraining. By the time of discharge from inpatient rehabilitation, George's tracheostomy had been decannulated. George was able to eat and groom with adaptive equipment after setup and he was able to verbally direct his care independently with increased time to communicate.

George lives alone in a multiple-level home. He worked full-time in a biochemistry lab as a technician. He is divorced and has partial custody of his son, Matthew, who stays with him on the weekends. George and his ex-wife get along fairly well, especially regarding the joint parenting of their son. George has been involved in a serious relationship with his girlfriend Mary for the past 3 years. They appear to be handling difficult situations well together in spite of potential strains on their emotional and physical relationship as a result of George's injuries. When George was not working, he enjoyed golfing, gardening, and riding motorcycles. While in inpatient rehabilitation, George started the process of exploring alternative and adapted leisure pursuits. However, he is still uncertain what he will do and wants to be able to do, especially after the halo vest is removed.

Upon completion of inpatient rehabilitation, the team (including George, his parents, and his girlfriend) decided that because of the level of care he required with limited support available, presence of the halo vest, and inaccessibility of George's home, it would be wise to pursue placement in an SNF. At the SNF, George could receive ongoing medical care, rehabilitation, and await the healing process of his cervical spine surgery with ultimate removal of the halo vest.

George is now transitioning for temporary placement at an SNF and has orders to be seen by CM, nursing, OT, PT, and SLP. He is able to eat and groom after setup with adaptive equipment and he is able to direct the rest of his care independently with increased time. He will need ongoing OT to facilitate improved independence in tasks, including upper body dressing and functional transfers. A rehabilitation physiatrist who makes rounds on all clients in the SNF will see him weekly. If indicated, George will also be able to meet with a psychologist once a week.

Analysis of Occupational Performance

Synthesis of Occupational Profile

George is a 47-year-old right-handed man in a halo vest with C5,6 AIS A tetraplegia. He lives alone, although he has a significant other who is supportive and interested in providing assistance for George if necessary upon discharge. He worked full-time in a biochemistry lab as a technician. He is divorced, but he remains deeply involved with his son and has an amicable relationship with his ex-wife. George's parents are older and live out of state; however, they remain emotionally supportive. He presents for OT 2 times per day, 5 times per week, to address improved communication and participation in his environment and ability to engage in his life occupations such as upper body dressing and functional transfers. Additional goals include prevention of potential secondary complications of brain and spinal cord injury. Although George, his significant other, and family members have learned and demonstrated improved understanding regarding George's spinal cord and brain injuries and their effects on his future function, they continue to need ongoing educational opportunities.

Observed Performance in Desired Occupation/Activity

Activities of Daily Living

Bathing: For bathing George is dependent. George is starting to be able to help a little with washing using a mitt attached around his wrist with velcro, but not enough to be at a maximal assistance level. He is able to direct his caregivers in completing bathing efficiently and safely.

Bowel and Bladder Management: Classified as having a C5,6 AIS A tetraplegia, George is unable to control his bowels or bladder without programs. George is now continent and regulated on a bowel program performed once daily. He requires medications and complete physical assistance to stimulate his bowels to evacuate. Because of his halo vest, and balance and strength deficits, he is unable to perform any parts of his bowel program at this time. Despite this, he can direct all parts independently with increased time. When in acute care, George had an indwelling Foley catheter for his bladder management. The Foley was removed during inpatient rehabilitation and George has been started on straight catheterization to empty his bladder every 4 hours. His halo vest makes it difficult for him to learn how to perform bladder management himself. He is wondering if he could use a mirror and some sort of brace for his hand so that he can regain some of his privacy and control over his body. George understands the importance of monitoring his fluid intake and output, but he still has difficulty making sure that he does not drink too much. He would like to be able to be straight catheterized less frequently than every four hours so that he can sleep through the night better.

Dressing: George is dependent for dressing tasks. He gets dressed from the bed level (i.e., while supine) to limit the burden of care on his caregivers. He has started to be able to initiate getting his arms into his sleeves, but because of the halo vest and decreased hand function he continues to require total assistance for upper body dressing. George is able to instruct his caregivers well in how to get him dressed efficiently.

Eating/Feeding: Setup is needed for all of his eating and feeding tasks. George is no longer on a modified diet and can drink thin liquids. He is unable to cut his food or open containers and packets, but he is able to eat using a hand-based universal cuff and bent utensils after a caregiver puts the equipment on his hand. He also uses a plate guard so that he can push food against the guard to get it onto his utensils. He is able to pick up a mug with an open handle and drink if the mug is half full; otherwise the mug is too heavy. George is able to instruct his caregivers well in how to set up his meal.

Grooming: He needs setup for grooming tasks. George is able to complete all parts of his grooming tasks (e.g., shaving, washing hands and face, brushing teeth, and combing hair) with adaptive equipment including built-up handles and a hand-based universal cuff. These tasks are still somewhat challenging because of the posts from his halo vest. He is able to perform his grooming while in his power wheelchair at an accessible sink. George is able to instruct his caregivers in how to set up the sink and equipment so that he can complete his grooming.

Functional Mobility: For overall functional mobility tasks, George ranges from being dependent to needing maximal assistance. He is able to help with rolling from side to side with the use of bed rails and maximal assistance. He is dependent with sitting up from supine or side lying. Because of discomfort and fear from his halo vest, George does not go into prone position. He is dependent using a portable mechanical sling lift or maximal assistance using a lateral transfer with a transfer board. George is able to lock out his elbows to maintain support of his upper body inconsistently, and he can push a little bit into his arms to help lift his bottom during the transfer. George is able to get into a power wheelchair that tilts back and he can stay upright at almost 90 degrees without getting dizzy or losing his balance for 2 hours at a time. He does get dizzy if he is transferred or is moved from supine to sitting too quickly. He is able to manage the goal post hand controls of the power wheelchair and drive indoors independently with occasional concerns for safety in tight spaces. He cannot manage the leg rests or armrests of the power wheelchair; he is dependent with these tasks. While in inpatient rehabilitation, George practiced manually propelling a rigid-frame manual wheelchair with a chest strap and push rims on level surfaces. He gets fatigued easily and has not been able to learn an effective way to propel that protects his shoulders.

Sexual Activity: George was sexually active and seriously involved with his girlfriend Mary before his injury. Currently he has not engaged in sexual intercourse because of his injury, precautions, and decreased understanding of adaptations to facilitate sexual activity. He is able to achieve an erection through touch, but the erection does not last long (i.e., less than 5 minutes). He is interested in receiving information about equipment and medication that might help with maintaining intimacy with Mary. Despite the fact that George cannot feel anything below his level of injury, he and Mary have experimented and found that George's shoulders and ears are even more sensitive to touch, particularly with kissing.

Sleep/Rest: Since his injury, George has been able to sleep better than he could while in acute care and inpatient rehabilitation, but still he gets awakened every 4 hours by nursing staff for repositioning and straight catheterization.

Toilet Hygiene: George is dependent for all toilet hygiene tasks. George is unable to manage his clothes or wipe himself. He is continent and regulated on a daily bowel program. He has a bowel movement once per day in the evening. He is being straight catheterized for his bladder management. In spite of his halo vest, George would like to start learning parts of straight catheterization that he can perform with help versus being out of control and reliant on others. He is able to verbally instruct caregivers in how to complete his toileting needs.

Instrumental Activities of Daily Living

Community Mobility: Before his injury, George drove cars and motorcycles. He is currently unable to drive because of residual physical and cognitive deficits. He is dependent on others for his community mobility. Although public transportation is accessible in his area, he remains unfamiliar with how to access it. He has not gone out on a day pass with his family, girlfriend, or friends, but he is interested in pursuing this option while at the SNF.

Health Management and Maintenance: George continues to have difficulties with medication management at this time. He is unable to hold his medications, although he can better recall what he is taking and when to take it. Before his injury, George went to his doctor annually and made sure to keep his hypertension and diabetes under control. George now is having difficulties with hypotension and is at risk for autonomic dysreflexia. He remains at risk for recurrent pulmonary emboli (PE) and pneumonia, but he continues to be treated prophylactically to prevent incidence of these secondary complications.

Home Establishment and Management: George is dependent for all home management tasks. George had been responsible for all home management, and he had especially enjoyed taking care of his lawn and garden. While in inpatient rehabilitation, George was able to participate in adapted gardening briefly, but he required increased physical and verbal assistance.

Meal Preparation and Cleanup: George was able to make simple, hot meals for himself and his girlfriend prior to the crash. While in inpatient rehabilitation, George was able to make a grilled cheese sandwich using adaptive equipment, with allowance for increased time and moderate assistance overall. He was able to clean up the cooking activity with maximal assistance. During the task, George was noted to burn his hand due to decreased sensation; he would benefit from further training to increase independence and safety.

Education

Formal Educational Participation: George graduated from college with a major in biology.

Work

Employment Interests and Pursuits: George was working full-time as a research technician in a biochemistry lab. His work demands frequent fine motor control, light lifting, and frequent communication.

Leisure

Leisure Exploration: George continues to be uncertain of leisure options that are available to people who have had a spinal cord injury. He participated in sessions with the therapeutic recreation specialist to learn about options for gardening and golfing, but he continues to demonstrate decreased awareness and ability to engage in exploration of leisure activity options. He is interested in learning more about his options and resources.

Leisure Participation: George enjoys gardening, golfing, and riding motorcycles. Although he has participated in therapeutic recreation sessions, George remains uncertain what parts of his leisure he can participate in as well as what other leisure options are available to him.

Social Participation

Family: George's parents are still living, but they live in a different town. They are older and, although emotionally supportive, they cannot provide support to George upon discharge. George still remains in contact with his ex-wife, particularly regarding decisions about their son, Matthew. George shares custody of Matthew, who spent weekends with George before the crash. George has been involved with Mary for the past 3 years. She is extremely supportive of him and is hoping to be able to help to take care of him after discharge and removal of the halo vest.

Peer, Friend: George has many friends who came to visit consistently while he was in the hospital; however, over time their visits have decreased. George has been distancing himself from his friends because of feeling like a burden and like a less able or less worthy person.

Factors Influencing Performance Skills and Patterns

Motor Skills

Posture: George's balance is still fairly poor in that he cannot sit unsupported without physical assistance, severe posterior pelvic tilt, and use of both arms. He cannot reach out of this base of support to engage in any other tasks without losing his balance. He is unable to accept any perturbations to his balance. George is able to sit on the side of a therapy mat with his hands out for support. He is able to transition between this position and throwing his arms behind him to support himself with minimal assistance to occasional contact guard assistance. He is able to tolerate sitting up in his power wheelchair with only a slight bit of tilt (i.e., 75 degrees versus 90 degrees of upright). He is able to tolerate sitting up in a wheelchair without physical assistance, but he needs a chest strap and seat belt to maintain upright and safe positioning. He no longer gets dizzy if sitting upright unless he gets up too quickly from lying down. His postural control remains limited further by his halo vest.

Mobility: As was stated previously, George's complete spinal cord injury leaves him unable to stand or walk. He is able to sit up in a wheelchair now without getting dizzy, with the exception of feeling orthostatic if he transitions into this position too quickly. He is able to manage driving a power wheelchair on level surfaces including navigating tighter spots with modified independence. He is able to access a tilt option on the wheelchair to perform pressure relief every 20-30 minutes. George is able to tolerate being in a standing frame or on a tilt table as long as care is taken with his halo vest; he cannot stand fully upright due to hypotension (less than 80/40 compared to his normal baseline of 105/60), but he can achieve a flexed position at 75% of full standing.

Coordination: George is right-handed. Because of his injury, he has decreased gross motor coordination and severely decreased fine motor coordination. His wrist extensors have been getting stronger and he has been learning how to use tenodesis function to pick up light and larger sized items.

Strength and Effort: George's muscle strength has increased, currently: shoulder flexion: 4+/5, shoulder abduction: 4/5, shoulder extension: 4+/5, elbow flexion: 4+/5, elbow extension: 1/5, supination: 3+/5, pronation: 0/5, wrist flexion: 1/5, wrist extension: 3/5, finger flexion: 0/5, finger extension: 0/5. George has started to have 1/5 movement in elbow extension and wrist flexion, but other than these movements he has none below his level of injury. He also does not have any increased sensation including presence of sacral sparing below his level of injury.

Energy: George has fair endurance, needing two rest breaks throughout a 30-minute therapy session. He is better able to control his secretions and does not become so fatigued when simply breathing. He rates his basic activities at below 11 using the Borg perceived exertion scale. His vitals are more consistently stable, with fewer episodes of hypotension. His baseline blood pressure is 105/60, his respirations are normal at 20, and his oxygen saturation on room air is consistently above 92 even with Borg perceived exertion of somewhat hard, 12 to 13 for more rigorous exercise or functional tasks. George still needs cues to pace his activities to account for his decreased energy level.

Process Skills

As a result of losing consciousness at the time of his crash, George initially demonstrated impairments in several areas of his cognitive function. Initially he was having difficulty with attention (select, alternating, and divided), memory, organization, sequencing, functional problem solving, and error identification. With intensive training and spontaneous healing, George is currently demonstrating mild to moderate, cognitive deficits specifically in his executive functions (e.g., planning, cognitive flexibility, attention/concentration, memory, organization).

Communication/Interaction Skills

George is still able to communicate his basic needs and discuss complex issues most of the time. He is better able to follow conversations and communicate his thoughts even if there are distractions (e.g., visual, auditory). While he was in inpatient rehabilitation, he had been practicing writing and drawing using a hand-based Wanchik's writer. He also started learning how to use a computer with a special trackball mouse and computer splint. He was also training his voice to a voice-activated computer program with good success. He remains interested in exploring options for using a voice-activated computer with hopes of learning skills for return to work or job retraining.

Habits and Routines

George has had complete disruption of his habits and routines. Not only does his physical condition make engaging in habits and routines challenging, but his continued mild to moderate cognitive deficits make difficult what used to be automatic. George has benefited from the structure of the inpatient rehabilitation program and is starting to re-establish some patterns regarding his morning and evening routines.

Factors Influencing Context(s)

Cultural

George is Caucasian. He values his family, especially his son. George also prides himself in his ability to work and is concerned that returning to his work as a biochemistry technician may be difficult unless there are accommodations that his boss can make.

Physical

George lives alone in an inaccessible home with many physical barriers to his current limitations. Most likely, he will need to explore alternative housing in a setting such as a group home.

Social

George's parents are still living, but they cannot provide much physical assistance because of their own health conditions and ages. George is divorced, but he stays in contact with his ex-wife and their son. George's girlfriend remains committed to supporting him throughout his rehab process.

Personal

George is a 47-year-old working right-handed man with a serious girlfriend.

Synthesis of Abilities and Deficits

Facilitators to Occupational Performance

George is motivated to get stronger and learn how to do things for himself again. He has an emotionally supportive social network, especially his parents and girlfriend. George has some motor return into his wrists and is learning to pick up things that are light and large so that he is better able to manipulate his environment. George's cognitive skills have been improving and he demonstrates mild to moderate deficits in higher cognitive abilities. George's girlfriend remains committed to learning how to provide physical assistance and hopes to be able to help to care for him at discharge when his halo vest is removed.

Barriers to Occupational Performance

Although George's family is supportive, they have limited ability to help with physical assistance or to provide 24-hour supervision if needed. His spinal cord injury at this point is complete, with only trace function in elbow extension and wrist flexion. He is physically unable to do any parts of his daily occupations.

Intervention

Intervention Plan

Collaborative Client Goals That Are Objective and Measurable

George has an anticipated duration of treatment at least 5 weeks, with an estimated frequency of OT 2 times per day for 30-minute sessions. By the time of discharge, George will perform the following:

1. Grooming with independence and adaptive equipment
2. Eating with independence and adaptive equipment
3. Upper body dressing with moderate assistance and adaptive equipment
4. Good understanding of equipment and positioning needs for increased participation in straight catheterization, at least at a maximal assistance level
5. Continued independent verbal direction of other aspects of care, including dressing, bowel program, toileting, and bathing
6. Actively participate in making decisions about discharge planning, including making necessary contact with accessible housing department and demonstrating good understanding of recommendations on home visit
7. Good understanding of education regarding spinal cord injury (e.g., pressure relief, skin care, autonomic dysreflexia, orthostatic hypotension, bowel/bladder, sexuality, neuroanatomy related to injury level) through ability to describe and answer questions pertaining to basic SCI education

By the time of George's discharge, Mary will demonstrate the following:

1. Good understanding of George's need for assistance/supervision

Discharge Needs and Plan

George wants to go home, with his girlfriend providing his care, but he is starting to realize that his house will be difficult to remodel; that making it accessible for a power wheelchair and hospital bed may be too hard. Mary will need to learn how to take care of George and be able to provide moderate to maximal assistance for all care except eating, grooming, and upper body dressing. Both George and Mary continue to benefit from extensive training regarding spinal cord and brain injury. If Mary cannot provide this level of care or his house cannot be realistically remodeled, it is likely that George will need to live in a group home setting. No matter what the final discharge plan is, George will continue to receive home health OT services.

Intervention Implementation

Therapeutic Use of Occupations and Activities

Occupation-Based Activities

Verbal direction of skin inspection, lower body dressing, bathing

Pressure relief

Facilitation of mobility

Toileting and bladder management

Upper body dressing

Functional transfers (bed, commode, shower, car)

Bed mobility

Communication with accessible housing staff

Purposeful Activities

Practice adaptive phone and call-light access

Practice transitional movements for transfers

Practice donning a shirt

Practice picking up adaptive equipment for bladder Management

Practice rolling from side to side in preparation for completing skin inspection and lower body dressing

Preparatory Methods

Biofeedback and neuromuscular electrical stimulation (NMES) to both arms

Orthotics and splinting for both hands

Practice fine and gross motor coordination

Stretching and strengthening programs

Positioning programs

Cognitive retraining

Consultation Process

Collaborate to determine the following:

Safest discharge setting

Best equipment for accessing nursing staff

Best equipment for increasing communication with family and friends

Best equipment and positioning for increased participation in occupations such as bladder management

Education Process

Provide family training about assistance and supervision needs

Reinforce education about spinal cord injury (bowel, bladder, skin, pressure relief, neuroanatomy of injury level, orthostatic hypotension, autonomic dysreflexia, and sexual function)

Reinforce education about brain injury (neuroanatomy and physiology, behavioral management, cognitive effects, influence of medications)

Reinforce nutrition counseling related to bowel management and healthy healing after spinal cord and brain injury

Provide education regarding choices for accessible housing

Intervention Review

Daily informal meetings set with OT to review progress, review treatment plan, and make modifications as needed.

Outcomes

Along with reviewing progress toward George's objective goals, therapy will continue to focus on his ability to resume participation in his roles of father, son, and boyfriend.

Questions

1. Your facility requires that you complete a mini mental state examination (MMSE) and geriatric depression scale on all of its residents. George scores 28/30 on the MMSE, but the GDS score is >5, indicating suspected depression. What do you do? Should you have any concerns that George's age does not fit the original age group for which the GDS was standardized?

2. George reports dissatisfaction and concern with the competency of staff regarding spinal cord injury. He provides examples of how he feels that his care has been neglected and he feels vulnerable. What would you do with this information?

3. How would you work to increase the comfort and competency of staff regarding care of persons with spinal cord or brain injuries?

4. To help carry over from session to session, you determine that it would be beneficial to have nursing staff help with setting George up appropriately. How would you propose to accomplish this so that staff members are informed and adhere to your recommendations?

5. Since George was admitted to the facility, 5 weeks have passed, which coincides with the potential removal of the halo vest. However, the doctor has already made rounds earlier in the week and will not be back until next week. What do you do?

6. Describe a session or two that addresses the goal of helping George participate in determining the best discharge setting, such as a group home.

7. What are some questions that he should have ready to ask staff members at the group home?

8. Given George's mild to moderate cognitive deficits, what compensatory strategies for organization might help him with setting up an appointment to go on a visit to the group home?

9. George's halo vest has been removed and a pressure sore is found beneath the vest. What can you do during your therapy sessions to help in his healing and education process?

10. When you are helping George with mobility and skin inspection of his healing pressure sore, you notice the start of a blister on his sacrum. George reports that although he has been performing pressure relief when he is up for the day, he still needs help to turn completely in bed, and no staff has been coming in when he calls for assistance. What do you do?

PART THREE

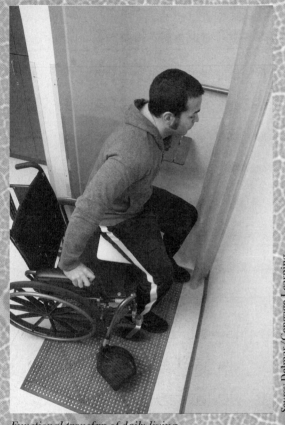

Functional transfers of daily living.

Inpatient Rehabilitation

Sandy

INPATIENT REHABILITATION

Level of Difficulty: Easy

Overview: Requires understanding of precautions related to hip replacement, including teaching use of adaptive equipment to a woman after hip replacement

Engagement in Occupation to Support Participation in Context(s)

Performance in Areas of Occupation: Spouse, mother, grandmother, professional career woman, and church member

Primary Impairments and Functional Deficits: Pain, generalized weakness, decreased understanding of how to incorporate hip precautions into daily activities

Context: Married professional 67-year-old woman near retirement

Occupational Profile

Sandy is a 67-year-old married woman who has severe osteoarthritis in her right hip. She has been less able to engage in daily exercise, and now the pain in her hip is limiting her ability to perform parts of her job such as standing for periods of time to present academic curriculum to her faculty members. She was found to be a candidate for a minimally invasive total hip arthroplasty. The surgery was uncomplicated; she stayed briefly in acute care to monitor her medical stability.

Sandy lives with her spouse in a two-level home with many stairs, although she is able to stay on the main level where she can sleep and have access to a bathroom. In order for Sandy to take a shower, she must be able to manage stairs. Downstairs, she has access to both a walk-in shower and a deep tub; she loves to take baths. Her spouse, who is retired, is the primary cook and does the main chores around the house.

Sandy still works full-time as an administrator for a local university. Her recent promotion to interim dean of the university brought increased responsibility and the reality that she travels out of town to be on the larger academic campus during

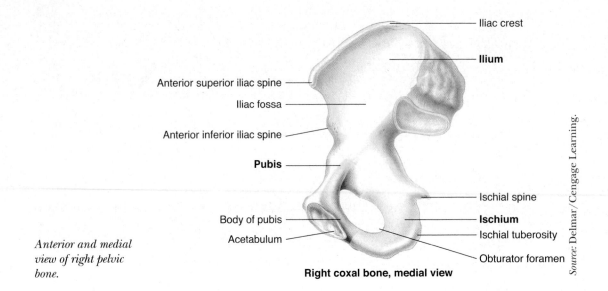

Anterior superior iliac spine

Iliac fossa

Anterior inferior iliac spine

Pubis

Body of pubis

Acetabulum

Iliac crest

Ilium

Ischial spine

Ischium

Ischial tuberosity

Obturator foramen

Anterior and medial view of right pelvic bone.

Right coxal bone, medial view

Source: Delmar/Cengage Learning.

the week. She plans to retire in the next 1–2 years or sooner if the university finds a permanent dean.

Sandy is active in her local church and attends regularly. Most of her friends in the area are from her church. Sandy also enjoys playing in the church bell choir, and when the bell choir performs she has to stand for at least 5 minutes at a time.

Sandy and her spouse have two grown children who are married and live out of state. Her eldest child, a son, has a 4-year-old son, and her youngest child, a daughter, just gave birth to a son a few months ago. Although her children live out of state, Sandy prides herself in trying to be involved as a grandmother.

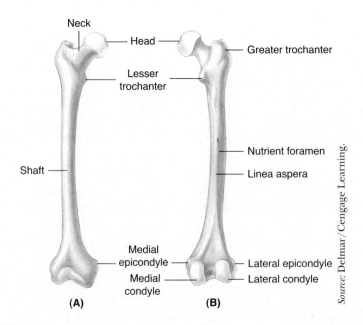

Neck

Head

Greater trochanter

Lesser trochanter

Shaft

Nutrient foramen

Linea aspera

Medial epicondyle

Medial condyle

Lateral epicondyle

Lateral condyle

The femur. A. Anterior view. B. Posterior view.

(A)   **(B)**

Source: Delmar/Cengage Learning.

According to the acute care notes, Sandy is functioning at a reasonable level except for needing additional time to work on lower body dressing, bathing, stairs, and identifying equipment needs for discharge to home. Furthermore, Sandy's spouse has received initial training, but he would benefit from additional reinforcement.

Sandy is now medically stable and has been evaluated by acute OT and PT and found to be an excellent candidate for a short 3- to 5-day stay in inpatient rehabilitation. She is being admitted to be seen by OT, PT, CM, nursing, and physiatry.

Analysis of Occupational Performance

Synthesis of Occupational Profile

Sandy is a 67-year-old married woman status post right total hip replacement. She is a professional career woman, spouse, mother, grandmother, and friend. She presents for inpatient OT to address equipment needs and use for resuming participation in the following areas of occupation: lower body dressing, bathing, and stair management.

Observed Performance in Desired Occupation/Activity

Activities of Daily Living

Bathing: She needs moderate assistance for bathing; she is able to wash her upper body but needs assistance to wash her right lower leg, foot, and bottom. She needs to sit on an extended tub bench for the majority of the time because of pain, decreased energy, and her hip precautions.

Dressing: She is independent with upper body dressing but needs moderate assistance with lower body dressing; she is able to get her underwear and pants onto her left leg but needs assistance to get them over her right leg, and she can then stand up and pull her pants up the rest of the way. She cannot put on her right sock or shoe without assistance.

Functional Mobility: She is modified independent for stand pivot transfers using a rolling walker. She can ambulate 100 feet, but she is unable to negotiate stairs at this time.

Toileting: She is modified independent with toileting; she is able to manage her clothing and wipe herself thoroughly with the assistance of a raised toilet seat and toilet safety frame.

Instrumental Activities of Daily Living

Community Mobility: Currently, Sandy is not able to ambulate outside because of decreased energy, pain, and fear of falling. The area around her home is hilly and extremely steep at some points. Before her hip surgery, she drove.

Health Management and Maintenance: Sandy is independent in managing her own medications and would like to be considered for self-medication while on the rehabilitation unit.

Home Establishment and Management; Meal Preparation and Cleanup: Although Sandy is capable of cleaning, cooking, and other home management, her spouse is primarily responsible for these occupations. Sandy is currently unable to perform light cleaning without pain or violating her hip precautions.

Education

Formal Educational Participation: Sandy completed education through postgraduate school, receiving a doctorate in education. She graduated with distinction.

Work

Job Performance: Sandy was a nursing professor at a local university for 15 years and has now been a nursing administrator for the last 15 years. She is well-respected by students, her staff, and her peers.

Retirement Preparation and Adjustment: Sandy has been preparing to retire for a while and plans to retire in the next 1–2 years. She tends to work intensely and is a little uncertain of what she will do in retirement. She is interested in volunteer opportunities. Sandy loves to travel to foreign places and to visit her grandchildren.

Leisure

Leisure Participation: Sandy has been less able to engage in leisure opportunities because of her current demanding work schedule. She enjoys singing, playing in the church bell choir, knitting, socializing with friends, and watching movies.

Social Participation

Community: Sandy is strongly connected with her church community and is an active member. She is less involved in politics but calls herself a moderate Democrat.

Family: Sandy has been married for over 40 years. She and her spouse have a good relationship. Sandy's children are grown and have their own families. She tries to be involved through visits and phone conversations in the activities and growth of her two grandchildren.

Peer, Friend: Sandy's friends are important to her and are mainly from her church community or work.

Factors Influencing Performance Skills and Patterns

Motor Skills

Mobility: Because of pain and generalized weakness, Sandy's mobility is decreased. She has tried to use a cane for ambulating, but she is unable to tolerate it at this point. She is able to get up and down from various surfaces without violating her hip precautions, but she wants to determine the best equipment to purchase for bathing/showering. She is unable to manage stairs.

Strength and Effort: After the hip surgery, Sandy demonstrates slightly decreased strength in her right leg, especially at her hip flexors, abductors, and extensors.

Energy: Sandy was less able to move around because of pain and generalized weakness before her surgery. As a result of this and the actual surgery, her energy is fair for her daily activities.

Process Skills

Knowledge: Sandy is able to state her hip precautions, but she is not able to incorporate them consistently into such tasks as lower body dressing or bathing.

Habits and Routines: Because of her hip precautions, Sandy's morning and evening routines related to lower body dressing and bathing have been disrupted.

Roles: Sandy is currently unable to return to work until she is able to perform community mobility and stand for prolonged periods of time. Both her work role and her ability to ring bells are affected.

Factors Influencing Context(s)

Cultural

Sandy has a strong Christian faith system.

Physical

Sandy's workplace requires much ambulating. At home, to get to her shower, she needs to manage a flight of stairs using one railing.

Social

Her spouse is supportive, although he is leery about seeing the hip incision or being responsible for any wound dressing changes. Sandy's church members and co-workers are already asking what they could do to help her as she recovers at home.

Personal

Sandy is a 67-year-old married, professional woman.

Synthesis of Abilities and Deficits

Facilitators to Occupational Performance

Sandy is able to verbalize her hip precautions. The hip surgery was uncomplicated and she is healing quickly. Sandy has a supportive spouse who is able to help her at home except for direct care of the hip incision. Sandy is able to ambulate household distances using a rolling walker. Last, but not least, Sandy has a background in nursing and a good understanding of the medical field.

Barriers to Occupational Performance

Sandy is experiencing pain and was generally weak before her surgery. To shower, she needs to be able to manage several stairs. Although she demonstrates the ability to state her hip precautions, Sandy has yet to learn how to use equipment to incorporate the precautions into lower body dressing and bathing.

Intervention

Intervention Plan

Collaborative Client Goals That Are Objective and Measurable

Sandy has an anticipated duration of treatment 3–5 days, with an estimated frequency of daily 90 minutes of OT. By the time of discharge, Sandy will perform the following:

1. Lower body dressing with modified independence and adaptive equipment
2. Bathing with modified independence and appropriate adaptive and durable medical equipment
3. Good understanding of hip precautions during daily routine, including light home management such as making a bed

By the time of discharge, Sandy's spouse will demonstrate the following:

1. Good understanding of equipment needs for discharge

Discharge Needs and Plan

Sandy is planning to return home. She needs to be able to learn how to use adaptive equipment to incorporate hip precautions. She needs to be able to negotiate stairs or she will have to have recommendations about sponge bathing. She will need to buy adaptive and durable medical equipment before discharge. Sandy's spouse is available to help her if needed and will benefit from additional education and training. It is anticipated that after leaving inpatient rehabilitation, she will not need any further OT.

Intervention Implementation

Therapeutic Use of Occupations and Activities

Occupation-Based Activities

Lower body dressing

Bathing/showering

Light home management

Purposeful Activities

Practice putting on socks with sock aid

Practice putting on underwear and pants with reacher

Practice unmaking and making a bed

Functional transfers

Practice standing while playing a bell

Preparatory Methods

Physical agent modalities: ice

Exercise: Calisthenics while standing

Consultation Process

Collaborating to determine the following:

> Safest equipment needs for lower body dressing and bathing
>
> Alternative bathing options if unable to manage stairs

Education Process

Client and family training of equipment recommendations

Education about hip precautions during daily activities

Intervention Review

Daily informal meetings set with OT to review progress, review treatment plan, and make modifications as needed.

Outcomes

Besides reviewing progress toward Sandy's objective goals, therapy will focus on her ability to resume participation in her roles as spouse, professional career woman, and church member.

Questions

1. What are Sandy's hip precautions? Besides lower body dressing and bathing, what are some other occupations in which Sandy will need to learn to incorporate her hip precautions?

2. How might your treatment be affected by changes to the surgical approach? That is, what if rather than a minimally invasive hip replacement Sandy had undergone either a posterior or an anterolateral approach hip replacement?

3. What are some additional purposeful activities that you would incorporate into treatment to help Sandy achieve her goals?

4. Would your approach to working with Sandy be any different because she is a nursing educator? Why or why not?

5. What are different methods that you might use to teach Sandy how to use adaptive equipment for putting on her clothes?

6. Write an example SOAP (Subjective/Objective/Assessment/Plan) note for a session with Sandy.

7. Describe your session with Sandy and her spouse regarding equipment recommendations for discharge.

8. You notice that Sandy seems not to care about being more independent with lower body dressing because it is so challenging. She keeps repeating that her spouse is retired and can help her. What do you say and do?

9. You arrive in Sandy's hospital room and find shortly after working with her that she is pale and complaining of lower energy and dizziness. Upon further questioning, you find that she reports that she has had black, tarry stools for the past few days. What do you do?

10. On the day before discharge to home, the OT asks you to go over recommendations to remove hazards that might increase the risk of falls in the home. What would be some of your discussion or demonstration points with Sandy and her spouse?

References

Gower, Dairlyn, and Bowker, Marcia. (2005). A Plumber and Golfer with Total Hip Arthroplasty, in *Ryan's Occupational Therapy Assistant: Principles, Practice Issues, and Techniques* (4th Ed.). Editors Karen Sladyk and Sally E. Ryan. Slack Inc. Thorofare, NJ.

James, Anne Birge. (2008). Restoring the Role of Independent Person, in *Occupational Therapy for Physical Dysfunction* (6th Ed.). Editors Mary Vining Radomski and Catherine A. Trombly Latham. Wolters Kluwer/Lippincott Williams & Wilkins. Baltimore, MD.

Maher, Colleen, and Bear-Lehman, Jane. (2008). Orthopaedic Conditions, in *Occupational Therapy for Physical Dysfunction* (6th Ed.). Editors Mary Vining Radomski and Catherine A. Trombly Latham. Wolters Kluwer/Lippincott Williams & Wilkins. Baltimore, MD.

Sladyk, Karen. (2005). Documentation, in *Ryan's Occupational Therapy Assistant: Principles, Practice Issues, and Techniques* (4th Ed.). Editors Karen Sladyk and Sally E. Ryan. Slack Inc. Thorofare, NJ.

Stephanie

INPATIENT REHABILITATION

Level of Difficulty: Moderate

Overview: Requires understanding of age-specific considerations in treatment along with clinical reasoning skills in the treatment of a teenager with a spinal cord injury

Engagement in Occupation to Support Participation in Context(s)

Performance in Areas of Occupation: Student, daughter, sister, part-time worker, peer, and girlfriend

Primary Impairments and Functional Deficits: Decreased strength, coordination, mobility, sensation, energy, decreased understanding of the effect of spinal cord injury

Context: Adolescent Caucasian girl

Occupational Profile

Stephanie is a 15-year-old girl who was a belted passenger involved in a single-vehicle rollover motor vehicle crash. She had short loss of consciousness after the crash. Cervical CT and MRI showed fractured cervical vertebrae (C5 and C6) and abnormal signal in the spinal cord at C5 and C6. There was edema in the cord, but there was no compression. She did not sustain any other injuries. To stabilize her neck and prevent further damage, a halo vest was placed surgically. She presents with decreased strength in her wrists and fingers (weaker and absent at times in right compared to left). She is able to move her left leg except for weakness in her ankle. She is not able to move her right leg except for trace hip extension and adduction. Her sensation is intact for pin prick on the right, but absent on the left. She has sustained a spinal cord injury and is a person with C5 SCI AIS C, tetraplegia with Brown Séquard syndrome.

Stephanie lives with her mother and her little sister, Beth. They live in a two-story home with four steps to enter with no rail. The lower level of the home has a full bath and bedroom, although Stephanie's bedroom is on the second floor.

Her parents are divorced and her father lives nearby. Although he provides little emotional or monetary support, Stephanie and Beth do spend every other weekend with their father. Stephanie's mother works full-time as a cardiac nurse.

Stephanie is a freshman in high school (typical grades are B+). She is active in drama, loves her science classes, and is good with Spanish. She has many friends and enjoys spending time with them. Besides socializing, Stephanie enjoys reading, watching movies, using computers, and ambulating.

Stephanie is saddened by the crash and her inability to feel and move the way she used to. She would like to be able to ambulate again or at least be as close to how she was before the crash. She shares that she is nervous about how people will look at her because she cannot move the way she used to, and moreover because she will have to wear her halo vest for at least 6 more weeks.

From the acute care reports, Stephanie appears to be able to urinate without difficulty, but she needs bowel medications to have a bowel movement. She is not able to stand at this time except in the parallel bars with two people helping. She cannot use her right hand.

Stephanie is now medically stable, has been evaluated by acute OT and PT, and is found to be an excellent candidate for inpatient rehabilitation. She is being admitted to be seen by OT, PT, therapeutic recreation specialists, case management, nursing, physiatry, and psychology services.

Analysis of Occupational Performance

Synthesis of Occupational Profile

Stephanie is a 15-year-old right-handed girl in a halo vest with incomplete tetraplegia. She is an active student, sister, daughter, friend, and girlfriend. She presents for inpatient OT to help her regain function to resume participation in her life roles with adaptations as needed. Stephanie and her family present with decreased understanding of her spinal cord injury and its effects on her current and future function.

Observed Performance in Desired Occupation/Activity

Activities of Daily Living

Bathing: She needs maximal assistance for bathing; she can wash and dry her right arm, her chest, and abdomen but needs help to wash and dry her left arm, front perineal area, buttocks, back perineal area, right leg and foot, and left leg and foot. The task is performed as sponge bathing because she is unable to transfer to a shower safely even with equipment at this time.

Bowel and Bladder Management: Stephanie is able to tell when she needs to urinate and does not need medication to control her bladder. She has problems with constipation and needs to take medications to help keep her bowels softer. Occasionally, she needs to have someone help to remove stool or perform digital stimulation (use of finger in circular motion at anus to start peristalsis reflex).

Dressing: She needs total assistance for getting dressed; she can instruct someone how to put on her bra, shirt, underwear, pants, socks, and shoes, but she cannot do any part of getting dressed.

Eating/Feeding: She requires minimal assistance for eating; she can eat 75% of her meal using her left hand and built-up utensils, but she cannot open containers and needs someone to cut her food up into small pieces.

Grooming: She needs moderate assistance for grooming; she can wash her face and brush her teeth with a built-up toothbrush, but she needs help to brush her hair and wash her hands thoroughly. She has not attempted to apply makeup, but she usually wears some.

Functional Mobility: She needs moderate assistance to scoot from her bed to a wheelchair with the armrest of the wheelchair removed. She is unable to stand up without the assistance of two people because her right leg is not strong enough to hold her and her left ankle twists.

Toileting: She needs total assistance for toileting; she is continent and able to go to the bathroom, but she needs help to get her clothes down, wipe after urinating or having a bowel movement, and pull her clothes back up.

Instrumental Activities of Daily Living

Care of Pets: At home, one of Stephanie's responsibilities is to feed her dog and take it for walks in the morning and evening.

Community Mobility: Stephanie is very active with her friends and enjoys ambulating around the mall. Currently, she is unable to stand without assistance and can do so only in parallel bars in the therapy gym. She cannot ambulate. Because of decreased hand function, she cannot propel a manual wheelchair at this point and is dependent on others for this mobility. Stephanie had planned to take driver's education this fall and to get her learner's permit.

Health Management and Maintenance: Before her car crash, Stephanie did not take medication. Now she is on medications for pain and to reduce constipation and increase ease of bowel evacuation. She was active in walking, but she did not participate in sports at school. She loves to eat junk food. She is unaware of how her nutrition might affect her now that she has a spinal cord injury.

Home Establishment and Management: Stephanie and her sister, Beth, have assigned chores at home such as keeping their rooms picked up, making their beds, and washing dishes after meals. Currently, Stephanie is unable to engage in any of these tasks.

Meal Preparation and Cleanup: Although Stephanie's mother does most of the cooking, Stephanie can make herself and her little sister snacks after they get back from school. Stephanie also enjoys making cookies to give to her friends and especially her boyfriend.

Education

Formal Educational Participation: Stephanie is in the 9th grade. She is currently taking a math class, a science class, a creative writing class, and a drama class. Her teachers have already figured out a system to send Stephanie her coursework by e-mail. She is having difficulty using the computer and is unable to write because of decreased strength and coordination, especially since she is right-handed.

Work

Employment Interests and Pursuits: Stephanie was working at a local grocery store bagging groceries and stocking shelves. She uses her money to be able to do things with her friends and her boyfriend. Because her father provides little financial support, Stephanie's mother has requested that some of the money Stephanie earns be put toward a college fund.

Leisure

Leisure Exploration: Although Stephanie does engage in leisure activities with her friends, she is interested in finding out more leisure options for her, especially if she needs to learn how to change the activities in order to pursue them.

Leisure Participation: Stephanie loves to be involved in anything dramatic. She is interested in trying out for a role in a play in the community playhouse. She loves hanging out with her friends to go shopping at the mall or go to movies. She frequently spends time text messaging her friends, but she cannot do this right now because her hands do not work well.

Social Participation

Community: Stephanie was an active 9th grader. She was working a few hours a week at a grocery store.

Family: Stephanie is very close to her mother. Although her little sister Beth annoys her, the two of them spend time playing together. Stephanie is not close to her dad, but she and her sister spend every other weekend with him.

Peer, Friend: Stephanie is very social with her friends. They love to spend time talking on the phone, text messaging each other, and going to the mall. She has a boyfriend and they like to go to movies, hold hands, and kiss each other. Because of her spinal cord injury, she might have issues with sexual dysfunction. She also is concerned about how her boyfriend and friends will interact with her while she has to wear her halo vest.

Factors Influencing Performance Skills and Patterns

Motor Skills

Posture: She has fair trunk balance in sitting and poor trunk balance in standing. She is unable to sit without her back supported.

Mobility: She is currently unable to ambulate and needs assistance to stand; she has decreased ability to support herself on her right leg, and her left ankle has a tendency to turn because of weakness and decreased sensation. She can move her left arm to reach for things and grasp items, but sometimes she drops them because she cannot feel things in her hand well. She cannot raise her arms over her head because of her halo vest and because of pain. Although she can reach with her right arm, she does not have strength to grasp anything. She does have increased ability to sense things on her right side. Although she is able to bend at her waist, she is limited by decreased balance and control, especially with her halo vest. She is limited in her ability to twist because of the vest. Stephanie cannot move her head or neck because of the halo vest plus her cervical precautions. Her mobility and other abilities are then affected because she has a decreased visual field. Furthermore, because she cannot move well, she is at risk for developing pressure sores.

Coordination: Stephanie's coordination is decreased on her left side because of decreased sensation, but she is able to stabilize and manipulate objects. She is not able to use her dominant right hand effectively at this time.

Strength and Effort: Stephanie's strength is decreased throughout her body, with her left side being stronger than her right side (3+/5 for left; 2/5 for right except for trace wrist movements and finger flexion for right). She demonstrates moderate loss in active range of motion in both her left and right arms.

Energy: When Stephanie first gets up out of bed, her blood pressure drops and she has difficulty with dizziness and nausea. She is supposed to wear an abdominal binder and knee-high compression stockings to prevent dizziness. Stephanie is able to tolerate an hour-long session of evaluation, but she needs frequent rest breaks. During the evaluation, Stephanie tends to try to do activities as quickly as she used to, but then she becomes exhausted.

Process Skills

Although Stephanie lost consciousness in the crash, all cognitive testing demonstrates that she is functioning within normal limits. She does demonstrate decreased understanding regarding her spinal cord injury and other medical concerns. However, she is receptive to information and asks questions appropriately. Stephanie's mother works in nursing and is able to understand medical information very well. She is interested in knowing all details about her daughter's care and recovery process.

Communication/Interaction Skills

Stephanie does not have problems with information exchange or engaging in or maintaining relations. She does, however, have difficulty with physical skills necessary for communicating effectively. Because of her halo vest, she has to turn her entire body to be able to look at people or else be seated directly in front of them. Although she used to use gestures to communicate, she is having difficulty now that she cannot use her arms and hands as well.

Habits and Routines

Stephanie still demonstrates automatic behaviors and occupations with established sequences in spite of her spinal cord injury.

Roles

Because of changes in her physical abilities, Stephanie is having difficulties in her roles as daughter, sister, friend, girlfriend, student, and part-time worker.

Factors Influencing Context(s)

Cultural

Stephanie is Caucasian. She values her connection to her family, especially her mother and sister.

Physical

Stephanie's home has many stairs to her bedroom and bathroom. Her classes at school are spread through out the entire building.

Social

Stephanie's mother is very supportive of Stephanie and her needs. Stephanie is strongly influenced by her friends, especially regarding her social routines.

Personal

Stephanie is a 15-year-old adolescent girl in the 9th grade. Her family is considered middle class although her mom works full-time and is a single parent.

Synthesis of Abilities and Deficits

Facilitators to Occupational Performance:

Stephanie is a young, healthy adolescent. She presents with an incomplete injury with excellent potential to regain some strength and control of her body. She thrives on interacting with people and enjoys communicating with her friends.

She is receptive to learning about her medical condition and is motivated to work in therapy to help resume her roles of daughter, sister, student, friend, and girlfriend. Stephanie's mother is very supportive of her daughter and has medical understanding because of working as a nurse.

Barriers to Occupational Performance:

Stephanie is in a halo vest to protect her neck from further damage, but this limits her mobility and ability to see things well. She has diminished sensation on her left side. She is right-handed and currently cannot use her right side much. The injury left Stephanie with pain in her neck and head. In the morning when Stephanie gets up she feels dizzy and nauseated because of low blood pressure. Stephanie has many steps at home and currently is just starting to be able to stand. Although Stephanie's mother is supportive, she works full-time and can take only limited family leave to help care for her daughter. Stephanie's dad has not provided emotional or financial support in the past.

Intervention

Intervention Plan

Collaborative Client Goals that are Objective and Measurable

Stephanie states that she wants to get back to doing her former day-to-day tasks.

Stephanie has an anticipated duration of treatment 3 weeks, with an estimated frequency of 90 minutes of OT treatment sessions at least 5 times per week. By the time of discharge, Stephanie will perform the following:

1. Grooming with modified independence and equipment as needed

2. Upper body dressing with moderate assistance and equipment as needed

3. Demonstrate good ability to resume student role with adaptations as necessary

4. Verbalize good understanding of basic spinal cord injury education (e.g., pressure relief, skin care, autonomic dysreflexia, orthostatic hypotension, bowel/bladder, sexuality, neuroanatomy related to injury level)

5. Independent verbal direction of care, such as bowel program, toileting, lower body dressing, and bathing

By the time of discharge, Stephanie's family and her peers will perform the following:

1. Demonstrate good understanding of Stephanie's need for assistance/supervision

2. Demonstrate good understanding of activity restrictions related to her spinal cord injury

Discharge Needs and Plan

Stephanie is planning to return home with help from her mother at a moderate assistance level for a few months until her mother returns to work full-time. It is anticipated that after leaving inpatient rehabilitation, she will continue with outpatient OT and possibly even hand therapy.

Intervention Implementation

Therapeutic Use of Occupations and Activities

Occupation-Based Activities

Total body dressing

Grooming

Eating/feeding

Simple meal preparation

Schoolwork

Play, leisure exploration

Purposeful Activities

Adaptive writing

Adaptive computer and phone access

Functional transfers

Practice throwing a ball to sister

Preparatory Methods

Sensory input to facilitate increased light touch and proprioceptive input

Biofeedback and functional neuromuscular electrical stimulation to both arms, especially right wrist/hand

Orthotics and splinting for right hand

Fine and gross motor coordination

Stretching and strengthening programs

Consultation Process

Collaborating to determine safest equipment needs for toileting and showering

Family training about best ways to have Stephanie and her sister interact

Education Process

Family training about assistance and supervision needs

Education about spinal cord injury (bowel, bladder, skin, pressure relief, neuro-anatomy of injury level, potential autonomic dysreflexia, sexual function)

Nutrition counseling, especially related to bowel management and healthy healing after spinal cord injury

Intervention Review

Daily informal meetings set with OT to review progress, review treatment plan, and make modifications as needed.

Outcomes　Along with reviewing progress toward Stephanie's objective goals, therapy will focus on her ability to resume participation in her roles as daughter, sister, friend, girl-friend, student, and part-time worker.

Questions

1. From Stephanie's occupational profile, what contexts support or inhibit her ability to achieve her goals for return to home?

2. What occupations and activities are successful or problematic for Stephanie?

3. How might your treatment approach change knowing that Stephanie is an adolescent? What might you do differently than you would with an adult or a pediatric client?

4. What would you do to incorporate Stephanie's friends into her rehabilitation program?

5. What are some potential concerns to be aware of regarding Stephanie's peers?

6. You are scheduled to do family training with Stephanie's mother and sister. What items would be critical to cover in preparation for discharge?

7. How would your approach to Stephanie change with the knowledge that the driver of the car in her crash was killed?

8. What would you add to your treatment approach if the driver and Stephanie had been found to be drinking? What referrals might you be responsible for making?

9. Stephanie's father calls you asking for information about her case. What do you do?

10. While Stephanie is in rehab, she needs to keep up with her schoolwork, but she is having difficulty with both writing and using the computer. What would you do to facilitate participation in her student role?

11. Stephanie has a new boyfriend. She is wondering how her spinal cord injury might affect her sexual function; how might you respond to her questions?

12. Considering Stephanie is an adolescent, how do you deal with discussions about sexuality?

13. Stephanie's mother is not present during the initial times that Stephanie divulges her questions about her sexual function. Do you have any responsibilities to share this information with her mother and, if so, how would you approach both the conversation and the education?

14. If Stephanie's spinal cord injury were not incomplete, she would be at increased risk for autonomic dysreflexia. She comes to your treatment session complaining of a headache. You notice that she is flushed from her shoulders up (above her injury level) and sweating profusely. What should you do?

15. You realize that Stephanie is meeting her current goals, therefore what would your discussion with the OT be regarding her goals and treatment plan?

References

American Spinal Injury Association (ASIA) and International Spinal Cord Society ISCOS. (2006). Standard Neurological Classification of Spinal Cord Injury patients. American Spinal Injury Association. Chicago, IL.

Atkins, Michal S. (2008). Spinal Cord Injury, in *Occupational Therapy for Physical Dysfunction* (6th Ed.). Editors Mary Vining Radomski and Catherine A. Trombly Latham. Wolters Kluwer/Lippincott Williams & Wilkins. Baltimore, MD.

Consortium for Spinal Cord Medicine. (2001). Acute Management of Autonomic Dysreflexia: Individuals with Spinal Cord Injury Presenting to Health-Care Facilities—Second Edition. Paralyzed Veterans Association. Washington, DC.

Ducharme, S.H. and Gill, K.M. (1997). *Sexuality after spinal cord injury.* Paul H. Brookes. Baltimore, MD.

Fike, M. Laurita, Pendleton, Karen, and Hewitt, Liane. (2005). A Telephone Repairman with Spinal Cord Injury, in *Ryan's Occupational Therapy Assistant: Principles, Practice Issues, and Techniques* (4th Ed.). Editors Karen Sladyk and Sally E. Ryan. Slack Inc. Thorofare, NJ.

Florey, Linda. (2005). A Teenager with Depression, in *Ryan's Occupational Therapy Assistant: Principles, Practice Issues, and Techniques* (4th Ed.). Editors Karen Sladyk and Sally E. Ryan. Slack Inc. Thorofare, NJ.

Paralyzed Veterans Association. (2000). Yes, You Can! A Guide to Self-Care for Persons with Spinal Cord Injury—Third Edition. Paralyzed Veterans Association. Washington, DC.

David

INPATIENT REHABILITATION

Level of Difficulty: Moderate

Overview: Requires understanding of treatment of pediatric population along with specialty treatment of burns

Engagement in Occupation to Support Participation in Context(s)

Performance in Areas of Occupation: Son, brother, and preschooler

Primary Impairments and Functional Deficits: Pain, decreased skin integrity, decreased range of motion, decreased ability to engage in meaningful play

Context: 2-year-old African-American toddler boy

Occupational Profile

David is a 2-year-old developmentally appropriate toddler who sustained deep partial-thickness burns on his lower body after being left in a hot bathtub unattended. The incident was an accident that happened while he was being cared for by a babysitter. To accelerate healing and minimize scarring, David underwent grafting to both legs.

David lives with his parents and his older brother and sister in a second-floor apartment.

David is enrolled in daycare where he is an active toddler and likes to play with other kids. He enjoys building things and running, and especially playing pretend by himself or with other kids.

David has been stabilized and now has issues regarding ongoing burn care in an inpatient rehabilitation setting. He is currently in the acute phase of burn management. He has been evaluated by acute OT and PT and found to be an excellent candidate for inpatient rehabilitation. He is being admitted to be seen by OT, PT, child life specialist, discharge planner, physiatry, and psychology.

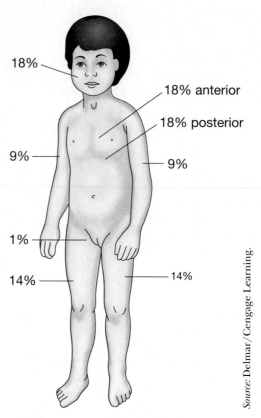

Source: Delmar/Cengage Learning.

The Rule of Nines in Measurement of Burn Surface Area Percentages.

Analysis of Occupational Performance

Synthesis of Occupational Profile

David is a 2-year-old African-American boy toddler who sustained burns on his lower body because of an accident in a bathtub. He is having difficulties with range of motion and mobility, wound healing, and psychosocial adjustment as they pertain to his ability to resume roles of son, brother, and preschooler. He is being admitted to inpatient pediatric rehabilitation to address these areas. Furthermore, David's parents present with decreased understanding regarding burn care management and how to modify tasks such as bathing and potty training considering his healing process and current limitations.

Observed Performance in Desired Occupation/Activity

Activities of Daily Living

Bathing: Since his injury, David has had help washing up by sponge bathing and has not attempted to take a bath. He appears to get upset at the mention of bath time.

Bowel/Bladder Management and Toileting: David had started potty training, but has been having increased frequency of accidents since his injury. Before his accident, he needed help with unfastening and fastening his buttons, snaps, and zippers, but was able to pull his pants down and up. He needed assistance to wipe thoroughly after pooping. He now needs increased help with pulling his pants down and up, and he needs total assistance to wipe, especially to make sure that his skin and dressings remain clean.

Dressing: Before his injury, David was able to take all of his clothes off, was able to put on his shirt, and could sometimes put on his pants except for fasteners by himself. He had not been able to put on socks or shoes without help. He is now having difficulties putting on his pants.

Functional Mobility: Because of pain and decreased mobility from healing burns and scar formation, David is having difficulty ambulating and running, but he is still able to do both activities. He used to love to bend down and get on the floor to build things, but now he avoids this because of pain and decreased range at his knees.

Play

Play Exploration: At preschool and at home, David spends much time with his stuffed animals imagining different scenes. He is starting to ask grownups and even his older siblings to tell him stories and he will sit still for a little while to listen to them. David likes stacking blocks and trying to build things. Since his accident, he is still interested in playing, but he is having difficulty getting into various positions because of pain and decreased range of motion.

Play Participation: David needs help learning to balance play, activities of daily living, leisure, and social participation. He has difficulty shifting from one area of occupation to the next, but he responds to time limits and reminders. David is able to get toys and other supplies for his playtime and can put them away after being asked.

Leisure

Leisure Exploration: Before his injury, David was involved in swimming and gymnastics lessons. He really loved the water and tumbling around. Since his injury, he is nervous about getting into the water. He fears tumbling around because of pain from his burns along with decreased mobility for rolling and squatting.

Leisure Participation: As was stated above, David needs help learning to balance play, activities of daily living, leisure, and social participation. He has difficulty shifting from one area of occupation to the next, but he responds to time limits and reminders. David is able to get toys and other supplies for his playtime and can put them away after being asked.

Social Participation

Family: David has developed strong relationships with his parents, sister, and brother.

Peer, Friend: David's mother organizes playtime for a few toddlers in the neighborhood. David enjoys playing with them and is learning to share his toys with them. David attends preschool and really likes being social with all of the kids.

Factors Influencing Performance Skills and Patterns

Motor Skills

Posture: David is not having difficulties maintaining his balance, although he does have loss of balance when attempting to squat to get blocks from the floor.

Mobility
Range of Motion: David is within normal limits for upper extremities; starting to have mildly reduced range at hip flexors, hip abductors; moderately reduced range at knee extension and flexion, and ankle dorsiflexion.

Coordination: David is not having difficulty with coordinating or manipulating items using his hands. However, his decreased range of motion and strength in his lower extremities affects his gross coordination.

Strength and Effort: David has normal strength for upper extremities and trunk; it is difficult to evaluate true lower extremity strength because of pain and decreased range of motion. He is having difficulty with lifting objects up from the floor into a standing position.

Energy: David's energy level remains unaffected by his injury.

Sensation

He is hypersensitive in the burned area except for being decreased for light touch and soft pinprick. All other areas are intact.

Skin Characteristics

Estimated Percentage of Body Surface Area Burn

Right Buttock: 2 1/2%

Left Buttock: 2 1/2%

Genitalia: 1%

Right Thigh: 6 1/2%

Left Thigh: 6 1/2%

Right Leg: 5%

Left Leg: 5%

Right Foot: 3 1/2%

Left Foot: 3 1/2%

Total Body Surface Area: 36%

Vascularity: The skin blanches with slow capillary refill.

Surface Appearance: The skin is wet with broken blisters.

Swelling: There is marked edema throughout the burned area especially around the feet and knees.

Height: It is difficult to measure the height or depth of the burned areas.

Pigmentation: Burn wounds on David's lower extremities and perineum are mixed red, waxy white.

Process Skills

Knowledge: David and his family demonstrate decreased understanding about his burn management. David's parents are eager to participate in his rehabilitation process.

Communication/Interaction Skills

David does not appear to have any interruption in his ability to convey his intentions or needs while coordinating social behavior in interacting with other people.

Habits and Routines

The primary habit that David had been working on was potty training. This has been interrupted by his injury.

Roles

So far, at age 2, David has established the following roles: son, brother, and preschooler. He is still able to participate in the first two roles, but he will not be returning to preschool until his body is a little more healed.

Factors Influencing Context(s)

Cultural

David's family has instilled strong family values. They come from an African-American background.

Physical

He and his family live in a second-floor apartment; other than that, there are no physical aspects of his environment that might pose a problem to him.

Social

David's strongest social influences come from his family and his preschool environment.

Personal

David is a 2-year-old toddler boy in preschool.

Synthesis of Abilities and Deficits

Facilitators to Occupational Performance

David has supportive parents who are invested in helping him to heal. David was and remains an active and healthy 2 year-old without previous issues of developmental delay. Although he has extensive burns, they are not currently infected and there are signs of healing already.

Barriers to Occupational Performance

David demonstrates decreased mobility, pain response, avoidance of certain activities, and psychosocial responses to his traumatic accident. Although his skin shows signs of healing, he remains at risk for infections.

Intervention

Intervention Plan

Collaborative Client Goals that are Objective and Measurable

David is unable to articulate clear goals. However, his family would like to bring him home and have him be able to return to playing and preschool.

David has an anticipated duration of treatment 2-3 weeks, with an estimated frequency of 90 minutes of OT treatment sessions at least 5 times per week. By the time of discharge, David will perform the following:

1. Put on socks, pants, and shoes in long sitting or circle sitting with minimal assistance
2. Increased hip, knee, and ankle range of motion as noted by tolerating playing with blocks in squatting position and prone for at least 10 minutes at a time

By the time of discharge, David's family will perform the following:

1. Good understanding of home program for stretching and positioning
2. Determine best setup for successful bathing at home with modifications as needed
3. Good understanding and return demonstration of burn care management, including dressing changes, massage, and donning/doffing burn pressure garment

Discharge Needs and Plan

David and his family are planning to take him home. Before they do so, they will need training in burn management and David will need to be free of infections and medically stable.

Intervention Implementation

Therapeutic Use of Occupations and Activities

Occupation-Based Activities

Play

　　Exploration play

　　Practice play

　　Pretend play

　　Games with rules

　　Constructive play

　　Symbolic play

Engage in activities with siblings

Total body dressing

Bathing

Grooming

Eating

Potty training

Functional mobility

Purposeful Activities

Practice picking up blocks from the floor

Practice pulling off socks in long sitting

Lie on platform swing in prone while tossing beanbags to his brother

Practice squatting to take off shoes

Brush teeth while stepping onto a stool

Work on climbing onto various surfaces of playground equipment

Preparatory Methods

Anti-contracture positioning

   Prone positioning

   Weights on thighs in supine

   Knee immobilizers

   Knee extension positioning and/or splints

   Prevent external rotation

   Position ankle at 90° with foot board or splint

Skin inspection and care

Desensitization

Scar management

   Massage

   Pressure therapy

   Fabricate and use specialized inserts

Range of motion (daily stretching routines and positioning programs)

Exercises

Transitional movements

   Pain management

   Psychosocial aspects of traumatic event

Consultation Process

Determine best method for returning to potty training considering scars and dressings with parents

Education Process

Educate parents about the following:

Range of motion, exercise program, splinting, and burn care program

Wear, care, and purpose of burn garment

Wound healing and tissue response to exercise and scar management techniques

Intervention Review

Daily informal meetings set with OT to review progress, review treatment plan, and make modifications as needed.

Outcomes

Along with reviewing progress toward David's objective goals, therapy will focus on his ability to resume participation in his roles as son, brother, and preschooler.

Questions

1. When working on an activity with David you notice that he is having more difficulties moving compared to previous days. Upon further exploration, you notice that he has increased pain, swelling, and decreased range of motion in his knees. What are some possible complications he might be having? What should you do?

2. You notice that David has ceased to gain range in his hips and knees which are limiting his ability to engage in play activities. You and the OT communicate this information to David's burn team. David ends up needing surgical release of his contractures. What is your role at this point?

3. What are some issues that David might have surrounding bath time now? How would you structure or grade treatment sessions to regain his comfort and willingness to participate in bath time again?

4. What additional activities might help David gain range in his lower extremities and ultimately allow him to return to his leisure and play areas of occupation?

5. Describe how your session teaching David's parents about wound care and activities to promote increased function would go.

6. Since David's burns are on his lower extremities, how would you explain your role as an OT contrasted with that of a PT?

7. David's parents are interested in resources about community programs available to David and themselves; what would you tell them?

8. What would be critical information to send along to David's preschool to facilitate smooth return to preschool?

Isaac

INPATIENT REHABILITATION

Level of Difficulty: Difficult

Overview: Requires understanding of cultural and spiritual needs of an Orthodox Jewish man who has suffered a stroke after elective knee surgery

Engagement in Occupation to Support Participation in Context(s)

Performance in Areas of Occupation: Educator, congregation member, spouse, and father

Primary Impairments and Functional Deficits: Decreased balance, coordination, range of motion, comprehension, expression, cognition

Context: Middle-aged Orthodox Jewish man

Occupational Profile

Isaac is a 50-year-old Orthodox Jewish man with past medical history significant for bilateral knee osteoarthritis. He was admitted to the acute hospital with severe aching and throbbing knee pain with left greater than right. He was unresponsive to conservative management with resultant decrease in functional mobility. He underwent an elective left total knee arthroplasty. Although there were no intraoperative complications, he developed acute onset of right-sided weakness, impaired speech, and cognition. MRI revealed an ischemic stroke.

Isaac is currently having limitations with his ability to return to his daily routine, not only because of limited strength and range of his left knee, but also because of neurological changes from his stroke.

He lives with a spouse and has six children (three of whom still live at home). Isaac's house is a split-level home. Their family maintains strict kosher practices according to their Orthodox background. They attend synagogue daily.

Because of his knee replacement, Isaac will wear a knee immobilizer on his left knee until he is cleared by PT for his ability to perform 10 independent straight leg raises. He is able to put as much weight as tolerated into his left leg, but he needs to avoid twisting or rotating his knee. Precautions related to his stroke are a high fall risk secondary to balance changes and medications.

Since his stroke, Isaac and his family have been very concerned about the prospect of their finances, as he is the only one in the family with an income. Isaac's

DIFFICULT

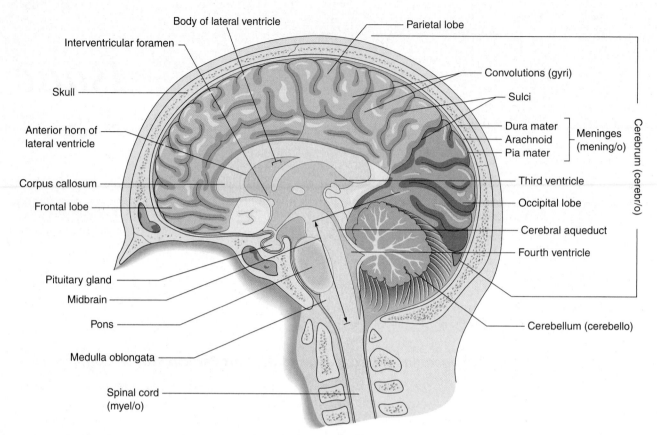

Interventricular foramen —
Body of lateral ventricle
Parietal lobe

Skull —
Convolutions (gyri)
Sulci

Anterior horn of
lateral ventricle —
Dura mater
Arachnoid — Meninges
Pia mater — (mening/o)

Corpus callosum —
Third ventricle

Frontal lobe —
Occipital lobe

Cerebral aqueduct

Pituitary gland —
Fourth ventricle

Midbrain —

Pons —
Cerebellum (cerebello)

Medulla oblongata —

Spinal cord
(myel/o) —

Cerebrum (cerebr/o)

Source: Delmar/Cengage Learning.

Section of the brain.

spouse is a stay-at-home mother and would be available to provide minimal physical assistance and 24-hour supervision.

Isaac is now medically stable and has been evaluated by acute OT, PT, and SLP and found to be a good candidate for inpatient rehabilitation. He is being admitted to be seen by discharge planning, nursing, OT, PT, physiatry, psychology, SLP, and TR.

Analysis of Occupational Performance

Synthesis of Occupational Profile

Isaac is a 50-year-old Orthodox Jewish man who had elective left total knee arthroplasty and then sustained a stroke with right-sided hemiparesis and cognitive deficits. He presents for inpatient OT to help him regain function to resume participation in his life roles with adaptations as needed. Isaac and his family present with decreased understanding of the effects of his stroke on his abilities. Furthermore, Isaac's spouse is uncertain that she will be able to provide more than minimal assistance to her spouse.

Observed Performance in Desired Occupation/Activity

Activities of Daily Living

Bathing: Isaac requires maximal assistance for bathing tasks; he is able to wash his right arm and chest but requires assistance with the rest. His balance is unsteady, so he is unsafe to sit unattended on a shower chair. Because of his religious beliefs, Isaac requests male caregivers.

Bowel and Bladder Management: Isaac has had urinary frequency and urgency. He is not always aware of when he needs to have a bowel movement and has had a few accidents since his stroke.

Dressing: Isaac requires total assistance to get dressed; Isaac has difficulty figuring out how to orient his clothes and puts things on out of sequence. He is not able to effectively help with getting dressed.

Eating/Feeding: Isaac requires moderate assistance for eating/feeding tasks; because of dysphagia, Isaac is on a modified diet. He has not been eating much and frequently needs encouragement, including being fed at times.

Grooming: For grooming tasks, Isaac requires maximal assistance. Isaac is able to wash his face, but he needs help to wash his hands, brush his teeth, comb his hair, and trim his beard.

Functional Mobility: Isaac requires total assistance for functional mobility tasks. He is able to help with rolling toward his right side, but he needs assistance to roll toward his left. He is able to help to go from sitting to supine, but he needs assistance lifting his legs up into bed. He requires assistance to go from supine to sitting. A sling is used to get Isaac out of bed and into his wheelchair or onto a commode because of his problems with balance, strength, and cognition. He is unable to propel his wheelchair at this time because of weakness and cognitive issues.

Toileting: Isaac requires total assistance for toileting. When incontinent of bowel, Isaac needs someone to help him manage his clothing and perform his hygiene. He continues to request male caregivers, especially for toileting.

Instrumental Activities of Daily Living

Community Mobility: Isaac had been driving, and he believes that after his knee stops hurting he will be able to resume driving without any troubles. He will need to rely on others for transportation in the community.

Financial Management: Isaac is responsible for all finances at home. Currently, this area needs to be assessed.

Health Management and Maintenance: Before his hospitalization, Isaac managed all of his medications, including those for hypertension and cholesterolemia. He currently needs his pills ground up and placed in applesauce. He cannot remember what medications he is taking or when he last took them. Besides issues with hypertension and cholesterolemia, Isaac is unaware of his other health risk factors and how to avoid them in the future.

Home Establishment and Management: Isaac's spouse is responsible for all duties inside the home. Isaac enjoys mowing the lawn and maintaining the landscaping around the house.

Meal Preparation and Cleanup: Isaac maintains strict kosher practices at home and has two separate kitchens, one to handle dairy and another to handle meat. His spouse is responsible for cooking. Their children help clean up after meals.

Safety Procedures and Emergency Responses: Isaac is a high fall risk because of his decreased balance, strength, and cognition. He is impulsive in his movements and unaware of safety issues surrounding him. When asked about emergency contact information, he is unable to identify whom to contact and what to say in case of an emergency.

Education

Formal Educational Participation: Isaac completed college-level coursework.

Work

Job Performance: Isaac works full-time at his local synagogue as an elementary school teacher. His job requires frequent communication and the ability to create lesson plans and carry them out effectively.

Leisure

Leisure Exploration and Participation: These areas are deferred to the therapeutic recreation specialists, although Isaac heard about a weekly outing that the hospital coordinates. He would like to go on an outing to his synagogue.

Social Participation

Community: Isaac is heavily tied to his congregation and his Orthodox beliefs.

Family: Isaac prides himself in being a disciplined father to his children, especially by instilling an understanding of the Orthodox Jewish traditions. He is a devoted spouse and prides himself on being the sole financial provider to his family.

Factors Influencing Performance Skills and Patterns

Motor Skills

Posture: When sitting unsupported, Isaac demonstrates decreased trunk control; he cannot maintain midline and pushes toward his weaker right side.

Mobility: Isaac is currently unable to ambulate. If he attempts to extend his left arm, he loses his balance. A mechanical sling is used to lift Isaac from one location to another; however, in physical therapy, he requires total assistance with two people to move from his wheelchair onto a mat. When Isaac tries to help during transfers he pushes himself hard toward his right side.

Coordination: Isaac's movements are not smooth and he cannot manipulate objects consistently. He needs cues and occasional hand-over-hand assistance to incorporate using his right hand in activities.

Strength and Effort: Isaac demonstrates slightly decreased strength in his left knee that may be related to decreased range of motion into flexion and extension. He is able to move all parts of his right side, but at a 3/5 grade strength. He exerts much effort to perform movements with occasional attempts to substitute other muscle movements to accomplish an activity.

Energy: Although Isaac is able to tolerate being in a wheelchair, he needs to rest every hour. When using his right arm and leg in activities, he loses control quickly as the activity continues or an exercise is repeated.

Process Skills

Energy: Isaac requires assistance to initiate and then pace himself during tasks. He is easily distracted and perseverates.

Knowledge: Isaac has difficulty figuring out what tools are necessary to complete his daily routine and life roles. He lacks the ability to figure out appropriate questions to help solve problems safely. Unfortunately, he also lacks insight into any potential safety concerns with his current abilities.

Temporal Organization: Isaac has difficulty initiating even familiar tasks like brushing his teeth. Once he finally gets started, he either perseverates on the task or becomes distracted and forgets the next steps.

Organizing Space and Objects: Isaac has difficulty finding things that he needs for various tasks. He needs step-by-step instructions and cueing. Once he has necessary objects for a task, he is unable to put them into a logical order without specific cues. Once he is finished with items for a task, he is unaware of what to do with them.

Adaptation: Isaac makes frequent, repeated errors, and he is unable to identify or correct them without specific cues.

Communication/Interaction Skills

Physicality: Although Isaac's right side is weaker and his balance is decreased, he still attempts to use his body when trying to communicate and interact with others, especially his spouse and children.

Information Exchange: Isaac has difficulty articulating ideas clearly both in thought and in actual speech production. Sometimes he needs to repeat himself to be understood and he tends to speak in short sentences. He is usually able to communicate his basic needs, but he has difficulty with more complex information. Isaac is having difficulty with recalling and reading the Jewish Bible, which is very distressing to him.

Relations: Isaac attempts to interact and relate with others, but he is easily distracted. He is less able to pick up on other people's reactions and requests.

Habits

Since his stroke, Isaac is demonstrating loss of useful habits. He cannot recall original habits that helped him in his daily routine and sometimes; because of perseveration, he tends to repeat habits such that he needs physical assistance and cues to stop them.

Routines

Isaac is having difficulty recalling familiar routines, but his spouse is extremely helpful in sharing details about them.

Roles

Isaac prides himself in the following roles: educator, congregation member, spouse, and father. Because of changes in his cognition, comprehension, expression, and physical abilities, he is having challenges in each role.

Factors Influencing Context(s)

Cultural

Isaac is an Orthodox Jewish man and maintains strict kosher practices.

Physical

Isaac's home is a split-level with a living room and kitchen on the entry level, bedrooms and bathroom on the upper level, a family room and bathroom on the lower level. It will be difficult to live on one level without managing stairs.

Social

Isaac has a strong and supportive family. His grown children have stated that they would be willing to come home to help their mother take care of their father, if necessary. Isaac's connection to his church and his work at the synagogue's school have provided him with good support from the congregation. The synagogue has been looking toward a fundraising event to help with medical costs and any equipment purchases or home modifications that Isaac and his family will need.

Personal

Isaac is a 50-year-old married working man with a college education.

Spiritual

Isaac's motivations and life purpose are to live out the word of his Orthodox Jewish traditions.

Synthesis of Abilities and Deficits

Facilitators to Occupational Performance

Besides osteoarthritis and a few risk factors for stroke, Isaac has been healthy. He is able to move all of his body in spite of decreased strength and coordination. Isaac's faith is strong in motivating him to return to his daily routines, especially work. Isaac's family and congregation are extremely supportive of his recovery and care.

Barriers to Occupational Performance

Isaac's stroke has resulted in changes in cognition, balance, comprehension, expression, and pushing behavior. He and his spouse are concerned about finances. Isaac's home is not accessible at this time. Although Isaac's faith is an asset, it also poses challenges in rehabilitation because the male caregivers he requests are less numerous in nursing and OT.

Intervention

Intervention Plan

Collaborative Client Goals that are Objective and Measurable

Isaac wants to be able to return to work, synagogue, and driving soon.

Isaac has an anticipated duration of treatment at least 3-4 weeks with an anticipated frequency of 90-minute OT treatment sessions at least 5 times per week. By the time of discharge, Isaac will perform the following:

1. Grooming with minimal assistance
2. Upper body dressing with minimal assistance
3. Lower body dressing with moderate assistance
4. Functional transfers (bed, toilet/commode, tub/shower, car) with moderate assistance to appropriate equipment
5. Good understanding of driving recommendations
6. 1-2 prevocational skills with moderate verbal cues

By the time of discharge, Isaac's family will perform the following:

1. Good understanding of equipment needs
2. Good understanding of need for assistance/supervision
3. Good understanding of home exercise program for strength, coordination, and cognition

Discharge Needs and Plan

Tentatively two discharge plans are needed. If Isaac's spouse and children are able to provide 24-hour supervision and moderate assistance for bathing, toileting, and lower body dressing, then the plan is to return home with temporary recommendations for living on one level until the home can be modified to accommodate a wheelchair. If the family is unable to provide this level of supervision and assistance, it will be necessary to switch to a temporary skilled nursing facility.

Intervention Implementation

Therapeutic Use of Occupations and Activities

Occupation-Based Activities

Total body dressing

Grooming

Eating/feeding

Toileting

Work

Purposeful Activities

Practice hemiplegia techniques for putting on a shirt

Practice trimming beard

Practice safe ways to get in and out of a walk-in shower equipped with grab bars and a shower chair

Read a passage from the Torah

Participate in pre-driving screen

Preparatory Methods

Neuro-reeducation

Sensory input to reduce pushing behavior and increase midline orientation

Biofeedback for upper extremity control

Fine and gross motor coordination

Coordination and strengthening programs

Cognitive retraining

Trunk balance

Knee range of motion

Consultation Process

Collaborate to determine the following:

  Safest equipment needs for toileting and showering

  Recommendations for home modifications

Education Process

Family training about assistance and supervision needs

Providing education about stroke and orthopedic conditions

Family training regarding home program for strengthening, coordination, and cognition

Providing education regarding return to driving recommendations and plan for further treatment options

Intervention Review

Daily informal meetings set with OT to review progress, review treatment plan, and make modifications as needed.

Outcomes

Along with reviewing progress toward Isaac's objective goals, therapy will focus on his ability to resume participation in his roles as educator, congregant, spouse, and father. Review of the plan and outcomes should also address need for switching to discharge plan of skilled nursing facility if Isaac's spouse determines she will be unable to care for her spouse at home.

Questions

1. You are a woman and have been scheduled to work with Isaac on a shower, but he has previously requested male caregivers; what do you do?

2. You notice when working with Isaac that he is focused on protecting his left knee when moving. How do you modify the setup of the task or provide cues to encourage increased functional use of his left knee?

3. You are waiting for Isaac to arrive in the therapy gym and find that he is late because he is trying to pray. What could you do to incorporate his interests and values into the therapy session?

4. You notice during a co-treatment session with you and the speech therapist that Isaac is refusing to eat. Knowing some of his cultural and spiritual preferences, what might account for this refusal and what could you do to improve his eating?

5. What additional purposeful activities might you introduce into therapy sessions to help facilitate achievement of Isaac's goals?

6. The OT asks you to perform a pre-driving screen and discuss the results with Isaac and his spouse. Although you have seen the screen performed, you feel that parts might require the evaluation skills of an OT. What would your discussion be with the OT to clarify this potential conflict in scope of practice?

7. Isaac's spouse asks you for advice regarding her ability to take care of her spouse at home. How might this conversation go? After you are done speaking with Isaac's spouse, you realize that she is leaning toward a skilled facility for his care rather than taking him home. Whom do you have responsibility to contact regarding the change in discharge plan?

8. You get a report from Isaac's nurses that they would like help with setting up a bed positioning program for Isaac. What would your recommendations be?

9. Because Isaac tends to forget to incorporate his right arm into daily tasks, but he has adequate strength, he is an ideal candidate for constraint-induced movement therapy. What activities would you set up for Isaac to promote increased functional use of his right side?

References

Logigian, Martha. (2005). A Businessman with a Stroke, in *Ryan's Occupational Therapy Assistant: Principles, Practice Issues, and Techniques* (4th Ed.). Editors Karen Sladyk and Sally E. Ryan. Slack Inc. Thorofare, NJ.

Woodson, Anne M. (2008). Stroke, in *Occupational Therapy for Physical Dysfunction* (6th Ed.). Editors Mary Vining Radomski and Catherine A. Trombly Latham. Wolters Kluwer/Lippincott, Williams, & Wilkins. Baltimore, MD.

George

INPATIENT REHABILITATION

Level of Difficulty: Difficult

Overview: Requires understanding of treatment of an adult with a dual diagnosis of spinal cord injury and brain injury with limited support system in an inpatient rehabilitation setting

---

Engagement in Occupation to Support Participation in Context(s)

Performance in Areas of Occupation: Full-time employee, adult son, father, and boyfriend

Primary Impairments and Functional Deficits: Decreased strength, coordination, mobility, sensation, energy, cognition, decreased understanding of the effects of spinal cord injury and brain injury

Context: Divorced adult Caucasian man with serious girlfriend

Occupational Profile

George is a 47-year-old right-handed man who sustained both spinal cord and brain injuries during a motorcycle crash. He was not helmeted and lost consciousness for at least 5 minutes. Upon admission to the trauma center, his GCS was 11. His blood levels did not demonstrate signs of alcohol or other substances. His trauma resulted in C6 level AIS A tetraplegia and moderate brain injury. Initially his cervical spine was surgically stabilized and then placed in a halo vest for 3 months. He also had a tracheostomy placed because of respiratory complications from the injury. His acute care course was complicated by a pulmonary embolism and pneumonia. He was treated with heparin and aggressive respiratory therapy.

George lives alone in a multiple-level home. He had worked full-time as a technician in a biochemistry lab. He is divorced and has partial custody of his son, Matthew, who stays with him on the weekends. George and his ex-wife get along fairly well, especially regarding the joint parenting of their son. George has been involved in a serious relationship with his girlfriend Mary for the past 3 years. When George is not working, he enjoys golfing, gardening, and riding motorcycles.

After a month in the acute care setting of the hospital, George is now medically stable. A physical medicine and rehabilitation consultation was requested, and George was found to be an ideal candidate for comprehensive inpatient

Thalamus

Cerebellum

Cervical plexus
C1–C5

Brachial plexus
C5–T1

Cervical enlargement

C1
C2
C3
C4
C5
C6
C7
C8
T1
T2
T3
T4
T5
T6
T7
T8
T9
T10
T11
T12
L1
L2
L3
L4
L5
S1
S2
S3
S4
S5

Lumbar plexus
L1–L4

Femoral nerve

Sacral plexus
L4–S3

Sciatic nerve

Lumbar enlargement

Filum terminale

Conus medullaris

Cauda equina

Filum terminale

Coccyx

Source: Delmar/Cengage Learning.

Spinal cord and nerves.

rehabilitation. George was also assessed by the acute care OT and PT team and found to be an excellent candidate for further rehabilitation. According to the PT and OT notes, George is having difficulty with tolerating sitting upright, but he is able to tolerate sitting up at a 45-degree tilt a couple of times per day of at least 45 minutes each. He demonstrates good potential to work up to tolerating the level of intensity needed for inpatient rehabilitation. He needs total assistance for all of his care and has cognitive deficits because of his brain injury. He is being admitted to inpatient rehabilitation, and he will be treated by OT, PT, therapeutic recreation specialists, case management, nursing, physiatry, and psychology services.

Analysis of Occupational Performance

Synthesis of Occupational Profile

George is a 47-year-old right-handed man in a halo vest with complete tetraplegia. Although he lives alone, he has a significant other who is supportive and interested in providing assistance, if necessary, upon his discharge. He had worked full-time as a technician in a biochemistry lab. He is divorced, but he remains deeply involved with his son and has an amicable relationship with his ex-wife. Although George's parents are older and live out of state, they remain emotionally supportive. He presents for inpatient OT to help him regain function to resume participation in his roles with adaptations as needed. George, his significant other (Mary), and family members present with a decreased understanding regarding his spinal cord and brain injuries and their effects on his current and future function.

Observed Performance in Desired Occupation/Activity

Activities of Daily Living

Bathing: His bathing tasks necessitate total assistance. Because of cognitive issues, George is having difficulty learning to instruct caregivers how to help him safely and efficiently. He needs maximal verbal and physical cues to understand what directions he should be providing to others.

Bowel and Bladder Management: Rated as an AIS A (Asia Impairment Scale), George is unable to control his bowels or bladder. George is currently incontinent of bowel, having bowel accidents a couple of times per day. He has not been started on an effective bowel program. He requires complete physical assistance to stimulate his bowels to move, along with medications to prepare his bowels for evacuation. He is also incontinent of urine, currently having a Foley, which he cannot manage. The Foley will be removed after a few days of determining his overall urine output (under 2000 ml) during a 24-hour period. When the Foley is removed, George will most likely need to have intermittent catheterization every 4 to 6 hours to empty his bladder. His halo vest makes performing bladder management himself nearly impossible at this time.

Dressing: Dressing tasks require total assistance. George gets dressed from a bed level to limit the burden of care on his caregivers and to limit episodes of dizziness. He does not know how to instruct his caregivers in the steps of dressing him.

Eating/Feeding: These tasks require total assistance. George is on a modified diet and nectar-thick liquids to prevent risk of aspiration, in part because of his inability to tuck his chin.

Grooming: George needs total assistance for grooming tasks; he cannot hold onto a toothbrush, comb, shaver, or washcloth at this point. He has difficulty sitting up for long before getting dizzy, so he has caregivers complete his grooming from bed level (i.e., while he is lying supine in bed).

Functional Mobility: He requires total assistance using a ceiling or portable mechanical sling lift because of best practice of safe handling on the rehabilitation unit. George is able to get into a tilt-in-space wheelchair, but he cannot stay upright past 45 degrees in it more than 5 minutes before getting dizzy or losing his balance. He can sit upright in the wheelchair for 45 minutes two times per day if he is at 45 degrees of tilt. He cannot propel the wheelchair at this time and is dependent on someone else to move him.

Sexual Activity: George was sexually active and seriously involved with his girlfriend Mary prior to admittance. Currently, he is unable to engage in sexual activity because of his injury, precautions, and decreased understanding of sexual function after a spinal cord injury. He is able to achieve an erection through touch, but the erection does not last long. He cannot feel anything below his level of injury.

Sleep/Rest: Since his injury, George has had difficulty getting a full night's sleep because of confusion and interruptions from staff coming in to turn him every two hours to prevent pressure sores.

Toilet Hygiene: For toileting tasks, George needs total assistance. He is unable to manage his clothes or wipe his bottom. George is currently incontinent of bowel a couple of times per day. He has not been started on a bowel program. He also has a Foley catheter and is unable to manage perianal care around the Foley.

Instrumental Activities of Daily Living

Community Mobility: Before his injury, George drove. He is currently unable to drive because of physical and cognitive deficits; he is dependent on others for his community mobility. Although public transportation is accessible in his area, he is unfamiliar with how to access it.

Health Management and Maintenance: George is having difficulties with medication management at this time. He is unable to hold his medications and he cannot recall what he is taking or when to take it. Before his injury, George went to his doctor annually and made sure to keep his hypertension (HTN) and diabetes mellitus (DM) under control.

Home Establishment and Management: These tasks necessitate total assistance. George had been responsible for all home management, and he had particularly enjoyed taking care of his lawn and garden.

Meal Preparation and Cleanup: Prior to the crash George had been able to make simple, hot meals for himself and his girlfriend. He currently needs total assistance with meal preparation and cleanup.

Education

Formal Educational Participation: George graduated from college with a major in biology.

Work

Employment Interests and Pursuits: George was working full-time as a research technician in a biochemistry lab. His work demands frequent fine motor control, light lifting, and frequent communication.

Leisure

Leisure Exploration: George is uncertain of leisure options available to people with spinal cord injuries. His current cognitive deficits prevent him from articulating specific interests in learning about his options and resources.

Leisure Participation: George enjoys gardening, golfing, and riding motorcycles. He is currently uncertain what parts of his leisure he can participate in or even what alternative activity options are available to him.

Social Participation

Family: George's parents are still living, but they live in a different town. They are older and, although emotionally supportive, they cannot provide physical support to George upon discharge. George still remains in contact with his ex-wife, particularly with regard to decisions about their son Matthew. George shares custody of Matthew, and before the crash Matthew would spend weekends with his dad. George has been involved with Mary for the past 3 years. She is extremely supportive and is hoping to be able to help to take care of George after discharge.

Peer, Friend: George has many friends who have been coming to visit consistently since his crash.

Factors Influencing Performance Skills and Patterns

Motor Skills

Posture: George's balance is poor. When working on his balance on a therapy mat, he needs moderate assistance to maintain short sitting, including needing to have his arms in extension and external rotation positioned behind him for increased support. If he tries to move one of his arms, he loses his balance backwards. He is unable to tolerate sitting up in a wheelchair without lateral supports, including a chest strap. He gets dizzy if sitting up past 45 degrees in the tilt-in-space wheelchair within less than 5 minutes. His posture is limited further by his halo vest.

Mobility: George's complete spinal cord injury (C 6 AIS A) leaves him unable to stand or ambulate. He is getting used to sitting up in a wheelchair, but he becomes dizzy if he gets up too quickly. He cannot propel the wheelchair. Most likely, he will be evaluated using a trial power wheelchair to see whether he can learn to drive it independently and safely. He will need to have a tilt option in the wheelchair to change his pressure every 20 to 30 minutes to prevent pressure sores as well as accommodate his decreased upright tolerance.

Coordination: George is right-handed. Because of his injury, he has poor gross motor coordination and severely decreased fine motor coordination. He has weak

(2/5) wrist extensors and may be able to start learning how to use tenodesis function to pick up items.

Strength and Effort: George's muscle strength is as follows: shoulder flexion: 4/5, shoulder abduction: 4-/5, shoulder extension: 4+/5, elbow flexion: 4/5, elbow extension: 0/5, forearm supination: 3/5, forearm pronation: 0/5, wrist flexion: 0/5, wrist extension: 2/5, finger flexion: 0/5, finger extension: 0/5. George does not have any movement, even 1/5, below his level of injury.

Energy: George has poor endurance. He gets fatigued just trying to breathe, particularly when secretions become loose and he has to try to cough them up. He needs rest breaks every 5 minutes during a 30-minute therapy session.

Process Skills

As a result of losing consciousness at the time of his injury, George is demonstrating impairments in several areas of cognitive function. He is having difficulty with attention (select, alternating, and divided), memory, organization, sequencing, functional problem solving, and error identification.

Communication/Interaction Skills

George is able to communicate his basic needs and discuss complex issues less than 50% of the time. He has difficulty following conversations and communicating his thoughts if there are distractions (e.g., dual tasks, noises). He is unable to write or type at this time because of his spinal cord injury.

Habits and Routines

George has had complete disruption of his habits and routines. Not only does his physical condition make it challenging to engage in habits and routines, but also his decreased cognition makes it difficult to recall certain tasks that used to be automatic.

Roles

Because of changes in his physical and cognitive abilities, George is having difficulties in his roles as son, father, worker, and boyfriend. He is uncertain what he will do without the use of his hands or being able to stand and ambulate.

Factors Influencing Context(s)

Cultural

George is Caucasian. He values his family, especially his son. George also prides himself in his ability to work.

Physical

George lives alone in an inaccessible home with many physical barriers to his current limitations.

Social

George's parents are still living, but because of their own health conditions and ages they are not able to provide much physical assistance. George is divorced, but he stays in contact with his ex-wife and their son. George's girlfriend Mary remains committed to supporting George throughout his rehabilitation process.

Personal

George is a 47-year-old working right-handed man with a serious girlfriend.

Synthesis of Abilities and Deficits

Facilitators to Occupational Performance

George is motivated to get stronger and learn how to do things for himself again. He has an emotionally supportive social network, especially his parents and girlfriend. George has some motor return into his wrists, which will permit him to learn how to pick up things and manipulate his environment better. George's girlfriend is currently committed to learning how to provide physical assistance and hopes to be able to help to care for him at discharge.

Barriers to Occupational Performance

Although George's family is supportive, they have limited ability to help with physical assistance or to provide 24-hour supervision if needed. George's cognitive dysfunction may make new learning more challenging. His spinal cord injury at this point is complete, and he is physically unable to do any parts of his daily occupations.

Intervention

Intervention Plan

Collaborative Client Goals that are Objective and Measurable

George states that he really wants to get the use of his hands back. He would also like to learn options for remaining intimate with his girlfriend.

George has an anticipated duration of treatment 6 to 8 weeks, with an estimated frequency of 60- to 90-minute sessions 5 to 6 times per week. By the time of discharge, George will perform the following:

1. Grooming with setup and adaptive equipment as needed
2. Eating with setup and adaptive equipment as needed
3. Directing other care verbally with modified independence, including dressing, bowel program, toileting, and bathing
4. Using the phone to dial 911 in case of emergency with adaptive equipment as needed
5. Verbalizing good understanding of basic spinal cord injury education (e.g., pressure relief, skin care, autonomic dysreflexia, orthostatic hypotension, bowel/bladder, sexuality, neuroanatomy related to injury level)

By the time of discharge, George's girlfriend, Mary will demonstrate the following:

1. Good understanding of George's need for assistance/supervision

Discharge Needs and Plan

George wants to go home to his house with his girlfriend providing his care. Mary will need to learn how to take care of George and be able to provide moderate to maximal assistance for all aspects of care except for setup with grooming and eating. Unfortunately, George's house is inaccessible, so they will have to discuss plans for remodeling the home or come up with a temporary plan. Both George and Mary will need to go through extensive training regarding spinal cord and brain injury. If Mary cannot provide this level of care or the home cannot be made more accessible, it is likely that George will need to go to a skilled nursing home temporarily or to a long-term care facility. Regardless of the final discharge plans, George will continue to receive OT services either at home or at a SNF.

Intervention Implementation

Therapeutic Use of Occupations and Activities

Occupation-Based Activities

Grooming

Eating/feeding

Verbal direction of skin inspection

Pressure relief

Purposeful Activities

Adaptive writing

Adaptive computer and phone access

Verbal direction of functional transfers

Practice using splint for eating breakfast

Practice using splint for brushing teeth

Preparatory Methods

Biofeedback and neuromuscular electrical stimulation

(NMES) to both arms/wrists

Orthotics and splinting for both hands

Fine and gross motor coordination

Stretching and strengthening programs

Cognitive retraining

Consultation Process

Collaborating to determine safest equipment needs for

toileting and showering

Education Process

Family training about assistance and supervision needs

Providing education about spinal cord injury (bowel/bladder needs, skin, pressure relief, neuroanatomy of injury, orthostatic hypotension, autonomic dysreflexia, and sexual function)

Providing education about brain injury (neuroanatomy and physiology, behavioral management, cognitive effects, influence of medications)

Ongoing nutrition counseling related to bowel management and healthy healing after spinal cord injury

Intervention Review

Daily informal meetings set with OT to review progress, review treatment plan, and make modifications as needed.

Outcomes

Along with reviewing progress toward George's objective goals, therapy will focus on his ability to resume participation in his roles of father, son, and boyfriend.

Questions

1. Describe a possible session to work on both functional skills and cognitive retraining. How would you decrease the level of assistance or cues that you are providing to George so that he remains successful in the session?

2. During your session to work on maintaining full and functional range of motion (ROM), you keep being interrupted by nursing's need to do various types of care. How would you approach the situation so that everyone's needs (George, nurse, OT) are met?

3. George's wrist control is improving, now allowing him to pick up smaller objects. How would you set up a session to work on practicing skills such as intermittent catheterization? You find that George's halo prevents him from seeing enough of his anatomy to be able to perform straight catheterization. What are some additional pieces of equipment that might allow George to see better?

4. George and Mary would like to know more information about sexual functioning after spinal cord injury. Describe how your discussion with them might go. How would you communicate to other team members (e.g., physiatrist, social worker, and/or psychologist) so that this knowledge gap is addressed appropriately?

5. While working with George you notice that he is complaining of a pounding headache and appears flushed from his shoulders up into his face. You take his blood pressure and find that it is 140/90. You suspect that he is experiencing autonomic dysreflexia. What steps will you take to avoid this life-threatening complication?

6. George reports that he smells as if he had a bowel movement before your session, but he really wants to stay to complete his strengthening program. What are your responsibilities and how would you discuss this with George and other team members?

7. After a few weeks of inpatient rehab, Mary realizes how much help George will need at discharge. You come into the room as Mary and George are discussing this realization and what to do. Describe what you would say and do.

8. How might the plan of care change now that it has been determined that George will need to go temporarily to an SNF, at least until his halo is removed?

9. What discharge information would you provide to the SNF regarding prevention of secondary complications of George's spinal cord injury?

PART FOUR

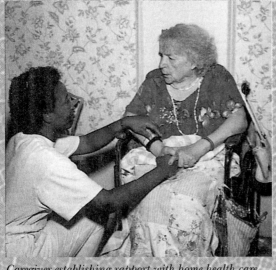

Source: Delmar/Cengage Learning.

Caregiver establishing rapport with home health care client.

Home Health Care

Gladys

HOME HEALTH CARE

Level of Difficulty: Moderate

Overview: Requires understanding of treatment of an elderly person regarding fall prevention in the home setting

---

Engagement in Occupation to Support Participation in Context(s)

Performance in Areas of Occupation: Widower, mother, grandmother, friend, and homeowner

Primary Impairments and Functional Deficits: Fear of falling, decreased balance, leg weakness, multiple medications, high risk of osteoporosis, limited engagement in activities

Context: Elderly woman who lives alone and has had recent history of falling

Occupational Profile

Gladys is an 80-year-old widowed woman who presents to her primary care physician with recent history of increased falls. An x-ray demonstrates presence of a healed wrist fracture along with suspected osteoporosis. The physician orders osteoporosis screenings with a bone density scan, which comes back positive for moderate to severe osteoporosis. Gladys is started on calcium replacement and it is determined that a course of occupational and physical therapy home health care would be beneficial for increasing her activity level while identifying additional risk factors for falls and establishing a fall prevention program.

Gladys lives alone in a townhome with three stairs to enter and no railing. Her main living area is on the first floor and then she can go down a flight of stairs with one railing to get to her bedroom and bathroom. She still drives, but she has limited herself to familiar areas and only at daytime, because she is uncomfortable with night driving and finding her way around in unfamiliar places. She enjoys visiting with friends and playing a weekly bridge game.

Gladys had been her spouse's primary caregiver until his death 10 years ago from myocardial infarction. Their three children live in the area and are able to help with groceries and occasional cooking.

Gladys is being evaluated for home health OT and PT to address identification of fall risk factors and establishment of a fall prevention program in the home and community.

Analysis of Occupational Performance

Synthesis of Occupational Profile

Gladys is an 80-year-old woman who presents with increased falls at home and was found to have several risk factors for medical complications including osteoporosis. She has decreased balance, endurance, fear of falling, vision, and understanding of risk factors and how to prevent falls. She is being seen for OT to determine further fall risk factors and establish a fall prevention program in the home to improve safety and ability to remain in an independent living situation.

Observed Performance in Desired Occupation/Activity

Activities of Daily Living

Bathing: Gladys requires minimal assistance for bathing and has a home health aide come to help her sometimes. Gladys prefers to take baths at night before getting ready for bed. She has fallen frequently when getting out of the tub/shower. Once she was unable to get out at all and had to wait until her daughter came by to check on her. She does not have any grab bars in the shower or non-skid strips on the bottom of the tub. Just outside of the tub, there is a bath mat that Gladys reports she has tripped on in the past.

Dressing: Gladys is able to complete total body dressing with independence and increased time. Gladys dresses herself, but she reports that sometimes she falls back onto her bed when she is putting on her underwear or pants. One time when she was stepping into her underwear, she fell forward and hit her nose on the floor. When ambulating in the house, Gladys prefers to wear slip-on slippers that have a smooth surface. When she goes out of the house, she still likes to wear her nicer clothes and has been known to put on dress shoes with heels. The shoes tend to have slippery or worn soles with narrow heels.

Functional Mobility: Gladys has difficulty ambulating and loses her balance frequently when talking or the phone ringing distracts her. She tends to reach for and hold onto furniture to get around.

Toileting: Gladys is independent with toileting tasks, although they take increased time. Gladys is able to manage her clothing and wiping with increased time, especially to get up from her low toilet into standing. She fell once adjusting her clothing after going to the toilet because her clothes had fallen around her ankles and she lost her balance reaching down to get them. There are no grab bars near the toilet.

Instrumental Activities of Daily Living

Community Mobility: Gladys reports that she has limited how much she ambulates outside of her home because of the fear of falling. Although she is able to ambulate 2 feet per second, she has difficulty ambulating 4 feet per second, which makes it difficult for her to cross city streets safely. She still drives, but she limits her driving to daytime, goes only to familiar places, and avoids roads with heavy traffic.

Health Management and Maintenance: Gladys is able to set out her medications for the week by herself using an enlarged pillbox. She needs to have caps on her pills that are easier to remove because of weakness in her hands. She takes multiple medications (i.e., more than four) throughout the day with the highest quantity in the morning. Although she routinely goes to her doctor for check-ups, she has ongoing troubles with hypotension, especially in the morning. After the loss of her spouse she became depressed, and she has been on antidepressant medication for the past several years.

Home Establishment and Management & Meal Preparation and Cleanup: Gladys limits her cooking because she does not enjoy cooking for just herself. She tends to make extra batches of meals that she can freeze and reheat later. She does love to bake cookies and have them on hand for her grandchildren for when they visit. Gladys reports that she once fell in her kitchen when she was trying to get something out of a low cabinet.

Education

Formal Educational Participation: Gladys received her college degree in elementary education. She prides herself on being a "lifelong learner" and still attends senior enrichment classes at the local senior center.

Work

Retirement Preparation and Adjustment: Gladys is a retired schoolteacher. She is able to manage financially because of her spouse's pension, life insurance, and her own retirement savings.

Leisure

Leisure Participation: Gladys enjoys knitting and crocheting while she watches television. Weekly she plays bridge with her friends. She enjoys having friends or family over for coffee and cookies.

Social Participation

Community: Although Gladys has been limiting her activities because of being afraid of falling, she does go to the local senior center at least twice a week to participate in various educational offerings.

Family: Gladys is a widow of 10 years. She misses the companionship of her spouse a great deal. Gladys's three children and seven grandchildren live in the area. Gladys's children take turns helping to get groceries, cook meals, and check on her, because she has been falling frequently.

Peer, Friend: Gladys plays bridge with friends weekly. She continues to entertain them occasionally at her house for coffee and cookies. Gladys expresses sadness that some of her older friends have passed away.

Factors Influencing Performance Skills and Patterns

Motor Skills

Mobility: Gladys answers "Yes" when asked the following questions:

1. Have you fallen in the past year?
2. Are you afraid that you might fall?
3. Do you frequently need to use your arms to get up out of chairs?

She tends to lose her balance when she is doing something at the same time as she is ambulating or moving. During the "Get up and Go" test, Gladys is able to rise from a chair with her arms folded, ambulate 10 feet, and return to the chair. It takes her more than 30 seconds to complete the initial test. When participating in a timed sit to stand test, she can get up fewer than 8 times in a minute.

Strength and Effort: Gladys demonstrates decreased grip strength and lower extremity strength, with her left leg being weaker than her right.

Energy: Gladys reports that she gets tired easily and sometimes becomes dizzy, especially if she stands up too quickly.

Vision: During a vision screen, Gladys demonstrates impairments in contrast visual acuity and contrast sensitivity, and she reports a history of untreated cataract in her left eye. These visual changes have been linked to being increased fall risk factors.

Sensation: Gladys demonstrates decreased proprioception, mildly decreased tactile sensitivity in her feet, and impaired vibration sensitivity in both legs. These factors have been linked to being risk factors for falls in the elderly.

Reaction Time: Gladys demonstrates moderately decreased reaction time, as tested by her ability to depress a switch in response to a stimulus of a light.

Postural Sway: When trying to stand still, a swaymeter indicates that Gladys has difficulty standing still on a medium-density foam surface. With her eyes closed, she has even more difficulty.

Process Skills

Knowledge: Gladys fears falling, because she has been falling during the past year. However, she is not aware of her fall risk factors and how to reduce them.

Habits and Routines

Although Gladys has set daily and weekly routines; she has been limiting her activities because of her fear of falling.

Roles

Gladys has been having difficulty with the loss of her spouse and of her long-term role as a spouse herself. She is a mother to three grown children and is a grandmother to their children. She continues to engage in her role as a friend, but she acknowledges sadness as her friends have gotten older and started to pass away.

Factors Influencing Context(s)

Cultural

Gladys prides herself on being independent. Cultural influences do not appear to be affecting her level of participation in her life roles.

Physical

Gladys lives alone in a townhome with many environmental barriers that may have contributed to her falls during the past year.

Social

Gladys enjoys spending time with friends, socializing over coffee and cookies, and playing bridge.

Personal

Gladys is an 80-year-old widow who lives alone.

Synthesis of Abilities and Deficits

Facilitators to Occupational Performance

Gladys is motivated to learn what is making her fall. She would like to learn how to improve her safety so that she can remain at home. Although she has several fall risk factors, she is cognitively intact and capable of learning and adhering to a fall prevention program. Gladys's children and friends are able to provide support by helping with cleaning, cooking, and running errands. They can also check in on her throughout the day by telephone and in person.

Barriers to Occupational Performance

Gladys demonstrates several fall risk factors: loss of balance, especially when talking and carrying items while ambulating; poor footwear; cluttered living space that makes use of a walker difficult; poor lighting, and vision especially at night when going to the bathroom; no grab bars, railings, or chairs, especially in bathroom; multiple medications; and self-restricted activity participation because of the fear of falling. Furthermore, Gladys was found to have moderate to severe osteoporosis and is at greater risk for injury if she continues to fall. Although Gladys's children and friends are supportive, she lives alone.

Intervention

Intervention Plan

Collaborative Client Goals that are Objective and Measurable

Gladys wants to learn ways to prevent future falls and remain living alone in her home. Gladys has an anticipated duration of treatment of 2 weeks with an estimated frequency of 2-3 sessions. By the time of discharge, Gladys will perform the following:

1. Demonstrate good understanding of fall risk factors and ability to adhere to a fall prevention program

2. Identify hazards in her home and be able to remove them to improve safety and reduce environmental risk factors for falls

3. Provide return demonstration of use of adaptive equipment and task modification for daily routines that improve overall safety

4. Demonstrate good understanding of home exercise program to increase activity tolerance in order to build bone mass

5. Learn and provide return demonstration of safe techniques to protect self in case of falling

Discharge Needs and Plan

Gladys wants to be able to remain living alone safely in her home setting. She will need to learn current risk factors for her increased falls and how to incorporate a fall prevention program, with a focus on removing hazards for falls in her home and building up her activity level to prevent complications from future possible falls.

Intervention Implementation

Therapeutic Use of Occupations and Activities

Occupation-Based Activities

Bathing

Lower body dressing

Toileting

Community mobility

Health management and maintenance

Home establishment and management

Meal preparation and cleanup

Safety procedures and emergency responses

Purposeful Activities

Practice getting onto floor and back up safely

Practice getting in and out of tub with equipment

Practice putting on clothing from seated position

Ambulate around block using four-wheeled rolling walker

Practice picking up items from floor using reacher

Perform home safety scavenger hunt

Practice ambulating without talking and while limiting distractions

Preparatory Methods

Endurance training

Strengthening

Flexibility training

Static and dynamic balance activities

Fall-recovery techniques

Visual compensation strategies

Consultation Process

Collaborate to determine the following:

Environmental hazards and how to remove them to prevent falls

Home modifications to prevent falls

Activities that can be incorporated into home exercise program to build bone mass and prevent worsening of osteoporosis

Collaborate with physician to determine medication management that reduces fall risk factors and promotes optimal function

Determine and provide training in equipment and activity modification to reduce falls

Education Process

Provide education and training on the following:

Realistic fall prevention plan

Safe ways to fall and protect from serious injuries

Use of personal help button to contact emergency response and use of cordless phone that can stay in walker basket when not in use

Intervention Review

Daily informal meetings set with OT to review progress, review treatment plan, and make modifications as needed.

Outcomes

Besides reviewing progress toward Gladys's objective goals, therapy will focus on her ability to resume participation in her roles as homeowner, mother, grandmother, and friend.

Questions

1. Write up a summary page that you can present to Gladys regarding identified fall risk factors to help improve her knowledge and awareness.

2. Write up a fall prevention program for Gladys that includes exercises to increase activity, environmental modification recommendations, and footwear based on her fall risk factors.

3. One of Gladys's fall risk factors is that she takes more than four medications. How would you facilitate reducing any unnecessary medications to control this risk factor?

4. The focus of your treatment session is going to be on environmental modifications to control external risk factors for falls. You have limited time, therefore how will you prioritize the session to have the biggest effect on fall prevention?

5. You arrive at Gladys's home and notice that she does not come to the door, yet you had confirmed with her earlier the time you would be arriving. You suspect she may have fallen; what do you do?

References

AOTA. (2006). Occupational Therapy and Prevention of Falls: Education for Older Adults,Families, Caregivers, and Health Care Providers. Retrieved April 19, 2009, from http://www.aota.org/Practitioners/Resources/Docs/FactSheets/Home/38513.aspx. AOTA Press. Bethesda, MD.

AOTA. (2007). Fall Prevention for People With Disabilities and Older Adults. Retrieved April 19, 2009, from http://www.aota.org/Consumers/Tips/Adults/Falls/35156.aspx. AOTA Press. Bethesda, MD.

Bogle Thorbahn, L.D., and Newton, R.A. (1996). Use of the Berg Balance Test to Predict Falls in Elderly Persons. *Physical Therapy Journal, 76,* 576-585.

Fall Prevention Center of Excellence. (2005). Basics of Fall Prevention. Retrieved April 19, 2009 from http://www.stopfalls.org/basics/using the search engine Google and key words "fall prevention and the elderly.

MN Chapter of APTA. (2008). Stand Up & Be Strong presentation at Combined Sections Meeting February 7. Retrieved April 19, 2009, from http://www.mnapta.org/subs/SUBS_csmpres6.pdf

Perry, J. (1992). *Gait Analysis Normal and Pathological Functions.* Slack, Inc. Thorofare, NJ.

Perry, J., Garrett, M., Gronley, J.K., and Mulroy, S.J. (1995). Classification of Walking Handicap in the Stroke Population. *Stroke, 26,* 982-989.

Shumway-Cook, A., Ciol, M.A., Hoffman, J., Dudgeon, B.J., Yorkston, K., and Chan, L. (2009). Falls in the Medicare Population: Incidence, Associated Factors, and Impact on Health Care. *Physical Therapy Journal, 89*(4), 324-332.

George

HOME HEALTH CARE

Level of Difficulty: Difficult

Overview: Requires understanding of treatment of person with dual diagnosis of spinal cord and brain injury in a group home setting

Engagement in Occupation to Support Participation in Context(s)

Performance in Areas of Occupation: Full-time employee, adult son, father, and boyfriend

Primary Impairments and Functional Deficits: Decreased strength, coordination, mobility, sensation, energy, higher-level cognition, medical stability (autonomic dysreflexia, orthostatic hypotension), decreased understanding of the effect of spinal cord injury and brain injury

Context: Divorced adult Caucasian man with a serious girlfriend

Occupational Profile

George is a 48-year-old right-handed man who sustained both spinal cord and mild brain injuries during a motorcycle crash 1.5 years ago. He was not helmeted and lost consciousness for at least 5 minutes. Upon admission to the trauma center, his GCS was 11. His trauma resulted initially in C6 AIS A tetraplegia and moderate brain injury. Initially his cervical spine was surgically stabilized and then placed in a halo vest for 3 months. He also underwent a tracheostomy because of respiratory complications from the injury. His acute care course was complicated by a pulmonary embolism (PE) and pneumonia. He was stabilized and then, after a month in the acute care hospital setting, transitioned to inpatient rehabilitation for 6 weeks, where the focus was on prevention of secondary complications of spinal cord injury, respiratory management, verbal direction of cares, education regarding spinal cord injury, and cognitive retraining. By the time of discharge from inpatient rehabilitation, the severity of George's brain injury had resolved to higher-level cognitive deficits. George was able to eat and groom with adaptive equipment after setup and he was modified independent in the verbal direction of his cares.

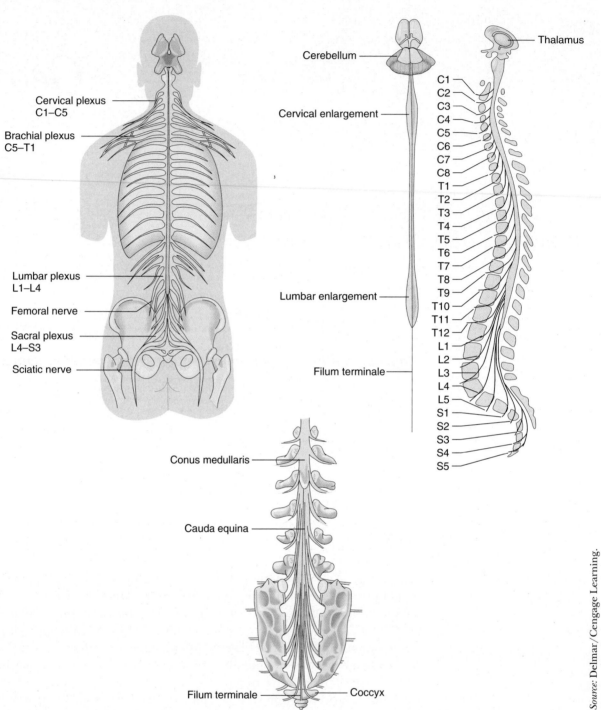

Source: Delmar/Cengage Learning.

Spinal cord and nerves.

Because his family was unable to provide the level of physical assistance required upon discharge from inpatient rehab, George went temporarily to an SNF for ongoing cervical healing and management of his halo vest. While at the SNF, he experienced complications of autonomic dysreflexia and development of sacral and ischial tuberosity pressure ulcers. He stayed at the SNF for almost a year. Now that his wounds have healed and his halo vest has been removed, George is transitioning to a group home. The group home is accessible for George's power wheelchair and he is able to take a bath/shower in a roll-in shower. He receives assistance from two personal care attendants, the first for 4 hours in the morning and the second for 3 hours in the evening. The group home does not have environmental control units, so George is limited by inability to control and interact with his environment.

George continues to be challenged by decreased independence and increased social isolation. He is being seen for initial evaluation and treatment in the home setting for OT with the focus on increased participation in occupations within his group home. George's physiatrist has ordered PT, CM, and psychology services in conjunction with home health OT.

Analysis of Occupational Performance

Synthesis of Occupational Profile

George is a 48-year-old right-handed man who sustained a traumatic spinal cord injury (SCI) with mild traumatic brain injury (TBI) during a motorcycle crash 1.5 years ago. His rehabilitation course has been long and complicated. He has been seen throughout the rehabilitation continuum to address increased independence and verbal direction of his daily routine. He is no longer immobilized in a halo vest, yet he still has residual higher-level cognitive deficits, specifically in the area of executive functions (e.g., planning, cognitive flexibility, abstract thinking, rule acquisition, and initiating appropriate actions and inhibiting inappropriate actions). George and his SNF practitioners felt that he would benefit from home health therapy services to improve independence with environmental accessibility, functional transfers, leisure participation, knowledge of resources available for community participation after spinal cord injury, and reinforcement of training related to spinal cord injury and assistance/supervision for George's personal care attendants (PCA).

Observed Performance in Desired Occupation/Activity

Activities of Daily Living

Bathing: He needs moderate assistance for bathing. George is able to instruct his PCAs how to bathe him efficiently and safely, but he would like to have help to instruct them in ways to facilitate his independence in bathing. George is able to take a shower in the roll-in shower at his group home seated on a high-backed rolling shower chair. He is able to help with washing his upper body and tops of his thighs although he continually drops his soap and washcloth.

Bowel and Bladder Management: Classified as having a C6 AIS A level of injury, George is unable to control his bowels or bladder. He is now on bladder and bowel programs and only occasionally has accidents. He requires complete physical assistance to stimulate his bowels, along with medications to prepare his bowels for evacuation. He is being straight catheterized every 6 hours so that his bladder can be emptied. George has had a few episodes of autonomic dysreflexia when his bladder was distended. George no longer has his halo vest and would like to start learning how to manage his bladder and bowel more independently if possible.

Dressing: George is dependent for lower body dressing and maximum assistance for upper body dressing. George gets dressed from a bed level to limit the burden of care on his PCA. He is able to roll from side to side with moderate assistance, which helps with getting his lower body dressed. He is able to direct his PCA well in how to get him dressed efficiently. He would like to try putting on his shirt once in his wheelchair to see if he is able to do it himself and therefore might be able to reduce the hours for needed PCA services.

Eating/Feeding: George can complete his eating/feeding tasks independently with increased time. He uses a plate guard, long straw, and universal cuff for eating. He is no longer on a modified diet and is able to tuck his chin if needed to prevent potential risk for aspiration. George would like to learn how to eat without adaptive equipment so that he can go out with his friends and family to restaurants without taking an entire backpack of equipment.

Grooming: George completes his grooming tasks with setup to stand by assistance. George can hold onto a toothbrush, comb, shaver, or washcloth to perform his grooming because of adaptations made by his previous OT. He is able to complete his grooming from a wheelchair level. He would like to reduce the number of adapted grooming supplies he uses in order to increase his independence and decrease the need for setup from his PCA. This would also alleviate any issues related to losing equipment.

Functional Mobility: George requires moderate assistance for bed-to-wheelchair transfers using a lateral transfer technique with a transfer board to level surfaces. He is able to manage transfers on unlevel surfaces with moderate/maximal assistance and increased need for the transfer board. Occasionally, George has difficulty locking his elbows during transfers. He also has difficulty leaning far enough forward and away from the direction of the transfer, which leads to losses of balance and increased need for assistance from his PCA or therapist. George is able to get into his power wheelchair and safely drive around both indoors and outdoors without assistance or issues with dizziness. He is also able to perform independent pressure relief using the tilt feature of his power wheelchair.

Sexual Activity: George was sexually active and seriously involved with his girl-friend Mary prior to the crash. He is able to achieve an erection through touch and takes medication to help it last longer. He cannot feel anything below his level of injury, but he notices that his ears and shoulders are highly aroused by Mary's touch. They have been able to experiment a little based on information provided by the psychologist and physiatrist.

Sleep/Rest: Since leaving the hospital setting, George is better able to rest and sleep without interruptions. He does not have access to frequent turning from staff at night so he tries to stay positioned on his sides to prevent further complications with his healed sacral sore.

Toilet Hygiene: George is dependent for all toileting tasks. He is unable to manage his clothes or wipe. George is now continent on regulated bowel and bladder management programs. He has help to complete a bowel program up on a padded commode once a day. His bladder program consists of being catheterized every 6 hours. He has tried to perform catheterizing since his halo vest was removed, but he needs to have a tenodesis orthosis to be more independent and successful.

Instrumental Activities of Daily Living

Community Mobility: Before his injury, George drove. He is currently unable to drive because of physical and cognitive deficits (although these issues are improving). He is dependent on others for his community mobility. He is able to take the bus and train near his group home by himself. His friends have expressed interest in being trained in transfers so that they can take George out with them.

Health Management and Maintenance: George is better able to manage his medications. Although he can pick up the various bottles, he cannot open them and is unable to handle the medications, so he needs assistance from his PCA or another staff member at the group home. Before his injury, George went to his doctor annually and made sure to keep his hypertension (HTN) and diabetes mellitus (DM) under control.

Home Establishment and Management: George is dependent for home establishment and management, except he has started to resume managing his finances with supervision from his father. George was responsible for all home management, and he especially enjoyed taking care of his lawn and garden.

Meal Preparation and Cleanup: George was able to make simple, hot meals for himself and his girlfriend prior to the accident. By the time of leaving the SNF, George was able to prepare simple hot meals with moderate assistance and adaptive equipment from a power wheelchair level. He was better able to complete cleanup with moderate assistance. He was working on following multiple-step instructions to improve his cognitive functions, including planning out the meals and safely completing the preparation and cleanup.

Education

Formal Educational Participation: George graduated from college with a major in biology.

Work

Employment Interests and Pursuits: George was working full-time as a research technician in a biochemistry lab. His work demands frequent fine motor control, light lifting, and frequent communication. He is becoming more aware that he might not be able to return to his work as a research technician unless his boss is willing to make accommodations.

Leisure

Leisure Exploration: George is still uncertain of leisure options that are available to individuals who have experienced a spinal cord injury. Now that his cognitive deficits are resolving, he is better able to participate actively in leisure exploration and is interested in learning about his options and resources.

Leisure Participation: George enjoys gardening, golfing, and riding motorcycles. He continues to be uncertain what parts of his leisure he can participate in or what other options are available, although he did work on adapted gardening with the therapeutic recreation and occupational therapists at the inpatient rehab center and nursing home.

Social Participation

Family: George's parents are living and are emotionally supportive, but because they are older and live in a different town they cannot provide physical support to George. George remains in contact with his ex-wife, especially regarding decisions about their son Matthew. George shares custody of Matthew; before the crash, Matthew would spend weekends with his dad. George has been involved with Mary for the past three years. Initially, Mary thought that she would be able to take care of George once he was discharged to home. Unfortunately, Mary decided that she could not handle the level of care that George would require. In spite of this, Mary and George remain involved and have been able to experiment sexually using some information that they learned from their psychologist and physiatrist. Because of George's adjustment to his injury and social isolation, his relationship with Mary is becoming strained.

Peer, Friend: George has been isolating himself from his friends, but a few of them still come around. They would like to be able to take him out, but they are uncertain how to transfer him in and out of their cars. They are also uncertain of good places to go with George that are accessible.

Factors Influencing Performance Skills and Patterns

Motor Skills

Posture: George's balance is fair. He is able to sit on the side of the bed and support himself with his elbows locked in an extended position. He is able to accept mild to moderate challenges to his balance, but he typically loses his balance backwards. He is able to reach out of his base of support, but he needs to anchor one arm around an armrest or the push cane to his power wheelchair. He is unable to tolerate sitting up in a wheelchair without support. He no longer gets dizzy when sitting upright unless he moves quickly from lying down to sitting up. He no longer has his halo vest and, as a result, is getting used to changes in his balance.

Mobility: As was stated previously, George's complete spinal cord injury leaves him unable to stand or ambulate. He is now getting around using a power wheelchair and only infrequently gets dizzy if he gets up too quickly. He is able to manage the controls on his wheelchair including the tilt feature, which he uses to perform pressure relief every 20 to 30 minutes. This is especially important for George since he developed decubitus ulcers on his sacrum and left ischial tuberosity while he was in the SNF. He is able to help with performing bed mobility and lateral transfers from wheelchair to bed with moderate assistance using leg and bed loops and a transfer board. He is sleeping in a hospital bed at this time to help with ease of providing his personal care.

Coordination: George is right-handed. His injury caused decreased gross motor coordination and severely decreased fine motor coordination. His wrist extensors are getting stronger, and he has been using tenodesis function to pick up larger, light objects.

Strength and Effort: George's muscle strength is as follows: shoulder flexion: 5/5, shoulder abduction: 4+/5, shoulder extension: 5/5, elbow flexion: 4+/5, elbow extension: 1/5, supination: 3+/5, pronation: 0/5, wrist flexion: 1/5, wrist extension: 3/5, finger flexion: 0/5, finger extension: 0/5. George has started to have palpable movements in elbow extension and wrist flexion, but other than these movements he does not have movement below his level of injury.

Energy: George has fair endurance, needing two rest breaks in a 30-minute therapy session. He rates most daily activities and exercises at a "somewhat hard" 12 to 13 on the Borg perceived exertion scale. He is better able to control his secretions and does not become so fatigued just breathing. He is able to pace his activities fairly well to account for his decreased energy level.

Process Skills

As a result of losing consciousness at the time of his injury, George initially demonstrated impairments in several areas of his cognitive function. Initially he was having difficulty with attention (select, alternating, and divided), memory, organization, sequencing, functional problem solving, and error identification. With intensive training and time to heal, George is demonstrating only mild, higher-level cognitive deficits; specifically in his executive function, including planning, cognitive flexibility, abstract thinking, rule acquisition, and initiating appropriate actions and inhibiting inappropriate actions.

Communication/Interaction Skills

George can communicate his basic needs and discuss more abstract issues. He is better able to follow conversations and communicate his thoughts even if there are distractions (e.g., dual tasks, noises). He is now able to dual tasks, follow 2- to 3-step instructions, and concentrate on a task for 30 minutes at a time. While he was in inpatient rehabilitation and at the SNF, he practiced writing and drawing using a hand-based Wanchik writer. He also started learning how to use a computer using a special trackball mouse and computer splint. He was training his voice to a voice-activated computer program with good success, and he remains interested in exploring options for using a voice-activated computer at the group home, with hopes of learning skills for return to work.

Habits and Routines

George has recently moved into his group home after being in an SNF. He has not been able to work on establishing successful habits and routines. His cognition is improving, but he reports feeling lost without the structure of the SNF setting.

Roles

George is doing better engaging in his roles of son and father, but he continues to be challenged in his roles as worker and boyfriend. Although he is able to manipulate larger items with his hands using tenodesis function, he remains uncertain what he will do without the use of his hands or being able to stand and ambulate.

Factors Influencing Context(s)

Cultural

George is Caucasian. He values his family, especially his son. George also prides himself in his ability to work, although he has become more despondent, believing that he will not be able to return to work because of the level of his spinal cord injury.

Physical

George has recently moved into a group home that is accessible via a power wheelchair. A ramp, an elevator, and equipment are available for a roll-in shower. Environmental control units (ECU) to access such things as phone, call lights, television, or computer are not present at this time.

Social

George's parents are still living, but they are not able to provide much physical assistance because of their own health conditions and age. George is divorced, but he stays in contact with his ex-wife and their son. George's girlfriend, Mary, has been having difficulties with the permanence of his disabilities and has determined that she is unable to step in as George's primary caregiver. Mary does remain committed to George emotionally, but the relationship is becoming strained.

Personal

George is a 48-year-old working right-handed man with a serious girlfriend.

Synthesis of Abilities and Deficits

Facilitators to Occupational Performance

George has made gains in his abilities since his original motorcycle crash. He is motivated to get stronger and learn how to do more parts of his daily routine, particularly regarding accessing more parts of his environment now that he has transitioned into a group home. His initial cognitive deficits have resolved to some degree and he has developed successful strategies to overcome residual deficits, although he continues to have difficulties with executive function skills. His parents, ex-wife, and son continue to provide strong emotional support. George is able to pick up various light objects and his trunk control has improved since his original injury. George is now living in an accessible group home and he has services of two PCAs for a total of 7 hours per day /7 days per week.

Barriers to Occupational Performance

Although George's family remains emotionally supportive; they have limited ability to help with physical assistance or to provide 24-hour supervision. George's cognitive deficits have improved, but he continues to have issues with higher-level deficits, especially executive functions (e.g., planning, cognitive flexibility, abstract thinking, rule acquisition, and initiating appropriate actions and inhibiting inappropriate actions). His spinal cord injury remains complete, and so his ability to perform all of his occupations without some level of assistance is challenging if not impossible. Although the group home is accessible with an elevator, chair lift, ramp, and roll-in shower, it is not accessible to enable George to do such things as managing the television, turning on and off the lights, and using a computer.

Intervention

Intervention Plan

Collaborative Client Goals that are Objective and Measurable

George would like to be able to access more things around the group home and make sure that his PCAs know how to take care of his needs completely.

It is anticipated that George will have a duration of 1 to 2 months with an anticipated frequency of three 1-hour sessions per week. By the time of discharge, George will perform the following:

1. Dress his upper body from wheelchair level with minimal assistance
2. Reinforce independent verbal direction of other aspects of care, such as lower body dressing, bowel program, toileting, and bathing
3. Use the phone to dial 911 in case of emergency and other key phone numbers with adaptive equipment as needed
4. Turn on and off lights and fan throughout group home using environmental control units (ECU) after setup
5. Use computer with voice activation and modified independence
6. Identify and use 2-3 compensatory strategies for tasks involving planning, cognitive flexibility, abstract thinking, rule acquisition, and initiating appropriate actions and inhibiting inappropriate actions

By the time of discharge, George's PCAs will perform the following:

1. Verbalize and provide return demonstration of good basic understanding of spinal cord injury (e.g., pressure relief, skin care, autonomic dysreflexia, orthostatic hypotension, bowel/bladder, sexuality, neuroanatomy related to injury level)
2. Demonstrate good understanding of George's need for assistance/supervision

Discharge Needs and Plan

George is now living in a group home that is wheelchair accessible. The PCAs and other staff members are familiar with working with clients who have cognitive deficits or developmental delays. They are less familiar with clients like George who have a spinal cord injury. The group home has not been equipped with environmental control units (ECUs) that would increase opportunities for George to engage with his environment more fully and independently. Home health OT services are ordered to address carry-over of skills and knowledge learned in previous settings. Finally, OT services will address completion of PCA training, verification of equipment needs, and best method for tasks such as transfers. Upon completion of home health care (HHC), George may be an ideal candidate for outpatient OT services.

Intervention Implementation

Therapeutic Use of Occupations and Activities

Occupation-Based Activities

Upper body dressing

Lower body dressing

Communication

Verbal direction of care

Pre-work skills

Purposeful Activities

Adaptive computer and phone access

Adaptive light and television access

Practice putting on a shirt

Practice long sitting and lower extremity management in preparation for participation in lower body dressing

Preparatory Methods

Neuromuscular electrical stimulation (NMES) to both arms/wrists

Fine and gross motor coordination activities

Stretching and strengthening programs

Cognitive retraining

Consultation Process

Collaborating to determine:

  Safest equipment needs and transfer techniques for toileting and showering

  Key areas at group home that can be accessed through ECUs

Education Process

PCA training about assistance and supervision needs Providing education and training about the following:

  Spinal cord injury (bowel, bladder, skin, pressure relief, neuroanatomy of injury, orthostatic hypotension, autonomic dysreflexia, and sexual function)

  Brain injury (neuroanatomy and physiology, behavioral management, cognitive effects, influence of medications)

  Use of environmental control units for group home setting

Intervention Review

Daily informal meetings set with OT to review progress, review treatment plan, and make modifications as needed.

Outcomes

Along with reviewing progress toward George's objective goals, therapy will continue to focus on his ability to resume participation in his roles of father, son, and boyfriend.

Questions

1. Plan out a session for training George to use an X-10 or other environmental control unit in order to increase his control over items in his room and other parts of the group home.

2. George has been able to get a voice-activated system attached to his power wheelchair and hospital bed, but he needs training to set up the system for his own voice. Describe the setup and training that you would complete to achieve a successful session where George can control his computer, DVD player, and television.

3. You notice that George is not ready and dressed for your session because his PCA did not show up for work today. What would you do to help George advocate for himself and make sure that he is not left in vulnerable situations such as this?

4. George reports that he had a pounding headache and goose bumps the other evening, and it took a while to convince his PCA of the importance of finding the potential source of these symptoms because of his risk and past with autonomic dysreflexia (AD). George asks for help to create a checklist that helps him instruct his PCAs when he is having an episode of AD. Design a day planner or task checklist that addresses training to deal with signs, symptoms, and treatment of autonomic dysreflexia.

5. You realize that George is becoming more withdrawn and appears to be isolating himself from his family, his son, and his friends. What might you do or suggest to address this increased isolation and potential depression?

6. During a training session with George and his PCA, you feel that they are not interacting in a safe and healthy way. What are your responsibilities and what is your response to the uncomfortable situation?

7. Design a functional treatment session to address improving George's cognitive skills in the area of executive functions (e.g., planning, cognitive flexibility, abstract thinking, rule acquisition, and initiating appropriate actions or inhibiting inappropriate actions).

8. George wants to work on transfers with his friends in and out of their cars. You know that one of the criteria for remaining a candidate for home health is that George be considered homebound other than leaving for medical appointments. What do you do?

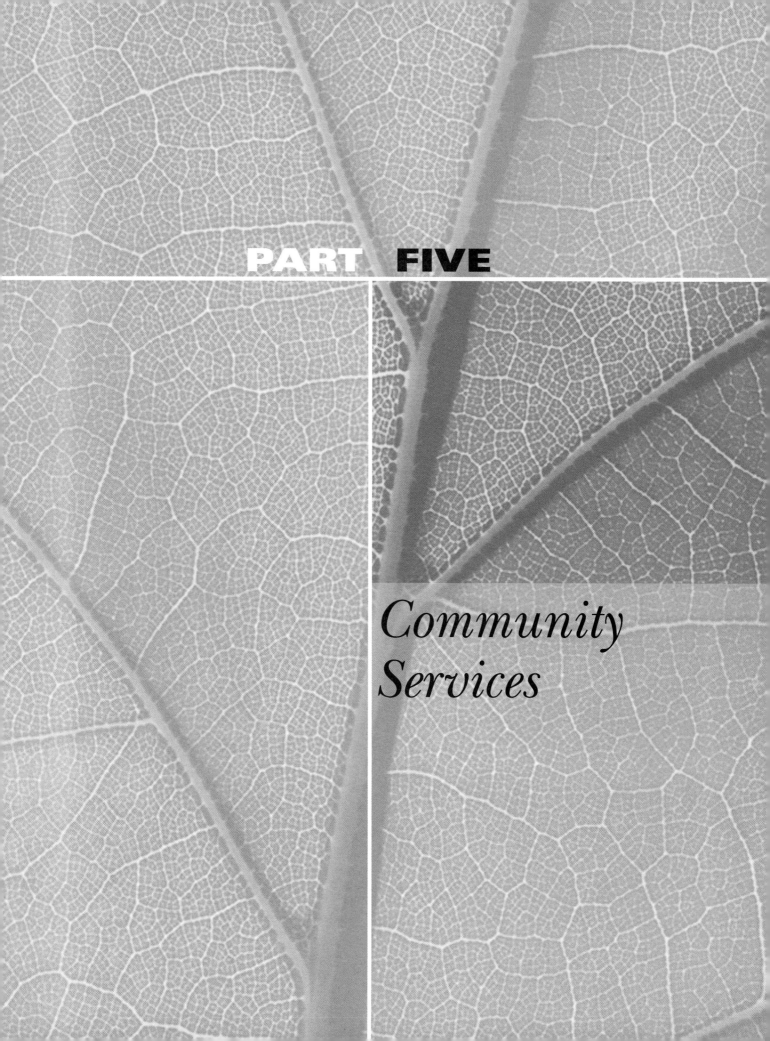

PART FIVE

Community Services

Fall Prevention and Osteoporosis Screening at Community Center for Elderly Day Program

COMMUNITY SERVICES

Level of Difficulty: Easy

Overview: Requires understanding of risk factors and treatment strategies related to fall prevention in a community setting of a geriatric day program

Engagement in Occupation to Support Participation in Context(s)

Primary Impairments and Functional Deficits: Presence of falls, decreased balance, decreased ability to perform timed sit to stand, decreased activity levels, fear of falling, decreased understanding of fall risk factors and prevention program

Context: Multiple geriatric clients in a community day program who have been identified as having moderate to high risk for falls

The following case study does not fit the format of the other cases regarding occupational profile and occupational performance. It involves working with a variety of clients in a geriatric day program in a community setting where fall prevention has been identified as a national safety goal. You and the OT are tasked with creating a fall prevention program for the center. The following questions are meant to help you in creating parts of the program.

Questions

1. What would be the key components of your fall prevention screening and why?

2. How would you run a session that helps clients create their own individual fall prevention plans?

3. Now that you have identified clients who are at moderate to high fall risk, design an hour-long group session to address improved skills for reducing fall risk factors.

4. You find that your screening indicates that a majority of the day treatment clients answer Yes to the question, "Are you afraid that you might fall?" What would you incorporate into your treatment sessions to address the emotional aspects of fall prevention?

5. You have determined that footwear can be a fall risk factor. Design a session that addresses discussion and intervention regarding improved footwear for the clients of the day program.

6. Describe a co-treatment session with nursing to address the high fall risk factor of multiple medications.

7. Set up a way to complete a remote home evaluation, without visiting clients' homes, so that you can collect more meaningful information about fall risk factors.

References

AOTA. (2006). Occupational Therapy and Prevention of Falls: Education for Older Adults, Families, Caregivers, and Health Care Providers. Retrieved April 19, 2009, from http://www.aota.org/Practitioners/Resources/Docs/FactSheets/Home/38513.aspx. AOTA Press. Bethesda, MD.

AOTA. (2007). Fall Prevention for People With Disabilities and Older Adults. Retrieved April 19, 2009, from http://www.aota.org/Consumers/Tips/Adults/Falls/35156.aspx. AOTA Press. Bethesda, MD.

Bogle Thorbahn, L.D., and Newton, R.A. (1996). Use of the Berg Balance Test to Predict Falls in Elderly Persons. *Physical Therapy Journal, 76,* 576–585.

Fall Prevention Center of Excellence. (2005). Basics of Fall Prevention. Retrieved April 19, 2009, from http://www.stopfalls.org/basics/

MN Chapter of APTA. (2008). Stand Up & Be Strong presentation at Combined Sections Meeting February 7. Retrieved April 19, 2009, from http://www.mnapta.org/subs/SUBS_csmpres6.pdf

Shumway-Cook, A., Ciol, M.A., Hoffman, J., Dudgeon, B.J., Yorkston, K., and Chan, L. (2009). Falls in the Medicare Population: Incidence, Associated Factors, and Impact on Health Care. *Physical Therapy Journal, 89*(4), 324–332.

COMMUNITY SERVICES

Level of Difficulty: Moderate

Overview: Requires understanding of treatment of elementary-school-aged child with autism in an integrated classroom of a school setting

Engagement in Occupation to Support Participation in Context(s)

Performance in Areas of Occupation: Son, brother, student, and peer

Primary Impairments and Functional Deficits: Decreased fine and gross motor function; decreased communication and interaction skills; decreased ability to regulate himself in response to stress and overstimulation; unwanted behaviors, including hitting head and being aggressive; and Brian, his parents, and teacher demonstrate decreased understanding of treatment options for successful inclusion in the kindergarten class

Context: 5-year-old kindergarten boy

Occupational Profile

Brian is a 5-year-old boy who is starting kindergarten in an inclusive classroom setting. He was diagnosed at age 3 with autism. He has participated in OT, SLP, and PT in the past. When he was younger, he was in preschool briefly, but he had difficulty with the poor structure, routine, and unclear rules. He would act out and hit his head. He interacted with others in the preschool aggressively or would isolate himself from others. His mother decided that it would be better to provide homeschooling and removed Brian from preschool.

Brian lives with his parents who are biracial (Chinese and Caucasian) and his two brothers and one sister. He does best at home with structured routines. He has difficulty with changes to his routine. He has been having difficulty interacting with his siblings without being too aggressive.

Brian enjoys anything to do with the weather and pirates. He can be found completely engrossed in his own play related to these topics and enjoys giving the weather report along with the evening news.

He is now demonstrating a need for increased academic and socialization opportunities. As a result, his parents have selected a kindergarten program that proves to be better structured than his former preschool. Unfortunately, Brian is still having difficulties, therefore his teacher and parents have decided to involve the school OT in order to determine the most successful approach for enabling Brian to participate well in his class. Brian is a good candidate for OT to address skills necessary for integration into kindergarten. The OT will also provide education to Brian's teacher, parents, and classmates regarding treatment strategies to continue once OT sessions are no longer needed.

Analysis of Occupational Performance

Synthesis of Occupational Profile

Brian is a 5-year-old boy with autism who is starting kindergarten in an inclusive classroom. He would benefit from sessions with the school OT to address deficits in fine and gross motor function, communication and interaction skills, ability to regulate himself in response to stress and overstimulation, and unwanted behaviors including hitting his head and being aggressive. OT will also help to improve Brian's, his parents', and the teacher's understanding of treatment options for successful inclusion in kindergarten class.

Observed Performance in Desired Occupation/Activity

Activities of Daily Living

Bathing: Brian does not like to be dirty. Brian does not like to take showers because of the pressure of the showerhead on his skin. He does like to take baths and create elaborate stories about pirates and their escapades on the sea.

Bowel and Bladder Management: Brian occasionally still has accidents and needs reminders to go to the bathroom at least two to three times per day. Other than reminders, he does not need help to manage his bowels or bladder.

Dressing: Getting Brian dressed for school is quite an effort because he does not like how clothing feels on his skin. He requests that all tags be removed from his clothes so that they do not scratch his skin.

Eating/Feeding: Brian is an extremely picky eater and has difficulty with certain textures of food.

Grooming: Brian has difficulty with the texture of toothpaste and getting him to brush his teeth is a struggle. He is able to brush his teeth best using an electric toothbrush and needs to have a set routine in the morning and at night to complete tasks such as grooming.

Functional Mobility: Brian likes to be fairly active, including running and jumping. He does have some difficulties with gross motor coordination. When stressed or overstimulated, he tends to pace around and jump.

Sleep/Rest: Brian does not have any problems with sleeping or resting, although after becoming overstimulated he benefits from being in a calm and quiet place. He does, however, have a rigid routine that he goes through in preparation for bed.

Toilet Hygiene: As stated before, Brian can lose track of time and needs reminders two to three times per day to go to the bathroom in order to avoid accidents. He does not need help with toileting.

Instrumental Activities of Daily Living

Health Management and Maintenance: Brian goes to his pediatrician for regular checkups. Since the age of 3, his parents and pediatrician have determined that Brian has autism. They have been collaborating on the best way to manage and treat him so that he can participate fully in school, play, and family roles.

Home Establishment and Management: Brian and his siblings have chores to complete at home. They are all to make sure to clean up their rooms.

Meal Preparation and Cleanup: Brian has a few chores as part of a structured routine at home. One of the chores is to help clean up dishes after dinner.

Education

Formal Educational Participation: Brian is just starting kindergarten. Before kindergarten, he was in preschool for a little while, but he had difficulty interacting appropriately with the other kids. The preschool did not have much structure, routines, or clear rules; Brian was removed and his mother then provided homeschooling. Brian's parents would like to get him involved with other children his age to help him learn various social and academic skills. Although the kindergarten class is better structured, the routines are still not clear enough for Brian to understand them. During circle time, he frequently gets up and paces or jumps and interrupts other classmates. Throughout the day, he can be found to have his ears covered by his hands and even hits his head on the table when highly stressed.

Brian enjoys counting anything and everything. He likes to be able to keep things in a specific order and organized. He likes to learn about anything to do with water where pirates might be sailing ships. He also loves to learn and talk about the weather.

Leisure

Leisure Exploration and Participation: Brian loves to collect things pertaining to pirates. He also likes to watch the weather television channel and practices being a weatherman. His parents bought him a weather map and pointer that he plays with every day. Brian likes to be able to jump and run in gym classes. He tends not to engage in leisure or play that involves interacting with others because he gets frustrated that he cannot always understand rules of their games and sports.

Social Participation

Family: Brian lives with his parents, two brothers, and one sister. They are having difficulty with some of Brian's behaviors and inability to interact without aggression.

Peer, Friend: Brian does not have many close friends, but his classmates make an effort to interact with him. Brian has difficulty relating to children his own age at times.

Factors Influencing Performance Skills and Patterns

Motor Skills

Posture: Brian does not have problems with postural control.

Mobility: As stated before, Brian loves to be active. He loves to run and jump. When stressed, Brian tends to pace.

Coordination: Brian has difficulty with gross motor coordination and can be awkward at times. He also has difficulty with fine motor coordination, including holding a pen, marker, or crayon for drawing and writing his name.

Strength and Effort: Brian does not have deficits in his strength; however, in his interactions with others, he is sometimes unaware of how strong he can be and has been known unintentionally to hurt other kids during play.

Energy: Brian has loads of energy and has difficulty sitting for longer than 10 minutes before needing to get up and move around or do something more physical.

Process Skills

Brian can become easily over stimulated, so that he has difficulty sitting still and working on an activity in his classroom. However, when working on something related to the weather or learning about pirates, he has good skills to sit still to process and incorporate new information.

Communication/Interaction Skills

Brian has difficulty talking and interacting with the other children in class. He cannot always understand their body language and facial expressions. He tends to keep to himself or go to the other extreme of interacting aggressively. When talking about pirates or weather, however, Brian is able to communicate fairly articulately.

Habits and Routines

To be able to get enough sensory and physical stimulation, Brian has been engaging in habits and routines that are disruptive to his overall learning and the other children in his classroom.

Roles

Brian is having difficulties participating successfully in his student role because of his autism and need for a certain level of active stimulation. He also has difficulty figuring out how to interact with his siblings without intense roughhousing.

Factors Influencing Context(s)

Cultural

Brian is biracial, Chinese and Caucasian. His father tends to speak to him in Mandarin Chinese to make sure that he becomes fluent in both Chinese and

English. His parents make every effort to celebrate and educate regarding their mixed cultural background.

Physical

Brian's classroom and overall school is laid out well and can be restructured to meet the needs of Brian and children like him.

Social

Brian tends to keep to himself and does not have any close friends his age other than his brothers and sister.

Personal

Brian is a 5-year-old Chinese/Caucasian boy who is starting kindergarten.

Synthesis of Abilities and Deficits

Facilitators to Occupational Performance

With the help of Brian's pediatrician, when he was 3 years old Brian and his parents were able to identify that Brian had autism. He is familiar with therapies such as OT and enjoys getting to play and feel less stressed when he attends therapy. Although Brian tends to isolate himself, he would like to interact and play with children in his kindergarten class. Brian's parents are eager to work on improving Brian's ability to interact with others and learning ways to decrease his aggressive interactions with his siblings. Brian loves anything to do with the weather and pirates. He loves to jump and run. Brian likes to organize and put things in order.

Barriers to Occupational Performance

Brian has difficulty regulating his behaviors when he is over stimulated or stressed. He demonstrates decreased fine and gross motor control. He has difficulty with situations that do not have structure, routine, or clear rules. He tends to isolate himself rather than try to communicate and interact with others. Brian has had limited success with integrating into a classroom setting, as demonstrated by difficulties in preschool.

Intervention

Intervention Plan

Collaborative Client Goals that are Objective and Measurable

Brian wants to be able to attend kindergarten and get along with the other children better.

Brian has an anticipated duration of treatment is 3-6 months with an estimated frequency of 2-3 treatment sessions per week. By the time of discharge, Brian will perform the following:

1. Be able to sit down for circle time, introduce himself, and stay engaged in circle time without disruptions at least 75% of the time

2. Participate in classroom activities for 40 minutes at a time before needing a sensori-motor diet break

By the time of discharge, Brian's teacher and parents will perform the following with Brian's input:

1. Identify four or five items to include in Brian's sensory diet that can be completed during the day

Discharge Needs and Plan

Brian, his parents, and his teacher would like his inclusion in the kindergarten class to be successful. Brian needs to be able to improve his communication, interaction, social skills, fine and gross motor skills, socially appropriate behaviors, and ways to decrease anxiety and overstimulation in order to participate fully in his classroom activities. He also needs to be able to learn less aggressive ways to interact with his siblings and other children. It is anticipated that Brian will need intense sessions of school-based OT initially and then will transition to periodic therapy intervention as new needs arise.

Intervention Implementation

Therapeutic Use of Occupations and Activities

Occupation-Based Activities

Practice Introducing self for circle time and sharing one item that you are interested in

Practice transitional activities

Fill out daily schedule using picture icons

Purposeful Activities

Structured play time

Adaptive techniques and strategies for writing

Preparatory Methods

Sensory diet

   Brushing and joint compressions

   Weighted blankets and deep pressure

   Swinging

   Bouncing on a therapy ball

   Ambulating on a balance beam

   Koosh balls and squeeze toys

   Music

   Headphones

Consultation Process

Collaborate to determine the following:

   Create a sensory diet that can be used during the day in the classroom

   Create best structure for the layout of the classroom, including visual schedules indicating when students need to move and the length of work periods

Set up and plan for transition activities to help with transition from one activity to the next

Set up color-coding system to help manage Brian's behaviors and class participation

Education Process

Provide education for the following:

To teacher about signs of high anxiety or difficulties that Brian may be having with sensory and emotional overload

To teacher about autism and its treatment

To students about autism and how best to interact with Brian

To teacher about the importance of consistent classroom routines to decrease anxiety and allow for increased independence in the classroom

Intervention Review

Daily informal meetings set with OT to review progress, review treatment plan, and make modifications as needed.

Outcomes

Along with reviewing progress toward Brian's objective goals, therapy will focus on his ability to resume participation in his roles of son, brother, and student, with primary focus on the student role and Brian's ability to remain engaged in his integrated classroom.

Questions

1. You notice that Brian tends to fidget and become more anxious when asked to try to write anything, including the alphabet. What might you suggest to the teacher to encourage Brian's participation in writing activities without increasing anxiety and unwanted behaviors?

2. Make a visual menu of appropriate behaviors that Brian can be prompted to demonstrate when he appears to be more anxious.

3. What would be some of the tasks that you might recommend Brian's teacher have in a separate "sensory area" in the classroom to which Brian is able to go when he is feeling more anxious or even when he has scheduled breaks?

4. What would your approach be regarding individual sessions with Brian that would address improved sensorimotor integration?

5. Brian's teacher approaches you to say that Brian is having difficulty socializing with the other kids. What might you recommend to improve his potential to learn appropriate socialization in his kindergarten class?

6. You notice that other children are having difficulty with Brian and his behaviors. What intervention could you suggest to help the students be more comfortable and understanding of Brian to achieve successful inclusion?

7. Part of the recommendation of the OT is to have a paraprofessional available in Brian's class, but there is also a need for a paraprofessional for three other students in separate classes. You find out that the school's budget is suffering and there is discussion of cutting back on the four paraprofessionals. Knowing about these possible cutbacks, what might you suggest in order to allow for continued success with inclusion for Brian and the three other children with special needs?

8. Based on the initial evaluation findings, what are Brian's interests and areas where he might have strengths in his classroom? How might you incorporate Brian's interests into increasing his successful participation in the classroom?

9. You know that providing structured choices is helpful for Brian and other kindergartners to be successful. What are some choices that you might recommend that the teacher establish throughout each day?

10. Brian has difficulty with recognizing and accepting changing from one activity to the next. How would you recommend that Brian be allowed transition time that clearly prepares him for the process of changing to the next activity?

References

Kluth, Paula. (2005). Supporting Students with Autism: 10 Ideas for Inclusive Classrooms. http://www.child-autism-parent-cafe.com/supporting-students-with-autism.html

Kluth, Paula. (2005). Teaching Autism Students in Inclusive Classrooms. http://www.child-autism-parent-cafe.com/autism-students-in-inclusive-classrooms.html

Rudy, Lisa Jo. (2007). Occupational Therapy and Autism: The Basics. http://autism.about.com/od/whatisautism/a/OTBasics.htm

Rudy, Lisa Jo. (2007). What Do Sensory Integration Therapists Do for Children with Autism? http://autism.about.com/od/treatmentoptions/f/sitherapydoes.htm

Sensory Diet: Autism Brushing Protocol Example. http://www.child-autism-parent-cafe.com/autism-brushing-protocol.html

The Autism Institute

MODERATE

COMMUNITY SERVICES

Level of Difficulty: Moderate

Overview: Requires understanding of treatment of elementary-school-aged child with autism in an integrated classroom of a school setting. More specifically requires understanding of how to provide education and training to new teachers and family members in a group setting

Engagement in Occupation to Support Participation in Context(s)

Primary Impairments and Functional Deficits: Decreased understanding of new teachers and family members regarding autism and its treatment strategies, especially in the context of integrated elementary school classrooms

Context: Variety of understanding and experience of new teachers and family members regarding elementary-aged children with autism

The following case study does not fit the format of the other cases regarding occupational profile and occupational performance. It involves working with new elementary school teachers and parents to provide training regarding work with children with autism. You and the OT are tasked with creating an Autism Institute that can be repeated annually and lasts for a two-day weekend. The following questions are meant to help you in creating parts of the Institute and thinking about the role of OT in the treatment of children with autism.

Questions

1. Create an outline of the key points to address when providing education to new teachers about working with children with autism.

2. Would your approach differ if your audience were to include parents of newly diagnosed children? Why or why not? If you answered Yes, how would the approach be modified?

3. One person participating in the institute appears to be monopolizing the floor; what do you do?

4. You know that you will have better results if you can incorporate interactive components into the institute versus a straight lecture format. Design some interactive breakout sessions.

5. Describe your session addressing how to help children with autism to work on social interactions.

6. How would you teach the group to identify strengths and areas to build rather than focusing on negative criticism or problem identification?

7. Set up a sample day planner for the children that might be useful for parents and teachers regarding communication of daily routine, rules, and expectations.

8. A participant expresses worry that including a child with autism in her class will take too much time away from the other students' learning opportunities; what would you say?

9. A parent reports that she is frustrated by repeated comments that her son will never be able to show emotions. What would you say to provide reassurance and suggest ways in which the parents and teachers might address other people's misconceptions about autism?

10. You know that sensory integration is a key part to successful treatment of children with autism. Describe how you would explain the common problems experienced by children with autism and ways that sensory integration can be used as an intervention.

References

Autisminspiration.com. Autism Information Handout. Retrieved October 16, 2008, from http://www.autisminspiration.com/public/122.cfm

Notbohm, Ellen. (2005). *Ten Things Every Child with Autism Wishes You Knew.* Future Horizons, Inc. Arlington, TX.

Sicile-Kira, Chantal. (2004). *Autism Spectrum Disorders: The Complete Guide to Understanding Autism, Asperger's Syndrome, Pervasive Developmental Disorder, and Other ASDs.* The Berkeley Publishing Group. New York, NY.

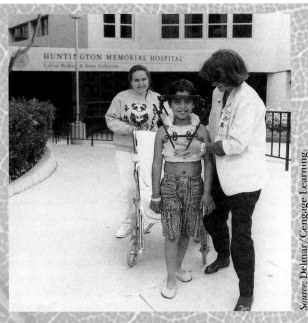

PART SIX

Source: Delmar/Cengage Learning.

Outpatient Rehabilitation

Wendy

OUTPATIENT REHABILITATION

Level of Difficulty: Easy

Overview: Requires understanding of treatment of Guillain-Barre and how to progress person toward return to work and driving given issues of decreased coordination and ataxia

Engagement in Occupation to Support Participation in Context(s)

Performance in Areas of Occupation: Businesswoman, spouse, and mother

Primary Impairments and Functional Deficits: Ataxia, decreased fine motor coordination, endurance

Context: Professional businesswoman

Occupational Profile

Wendy is a 55-year-old left-handed businesswoman who was in her usual state of good health when she developed flu-like symptoms including back pain. After a number of sick days off from work, she noticed that she was beginning to feel weak all over, but mainly in her legs, arms, and face. Wendy noticed intermittent tingling and numbness in her face and lips. She was also having difficulty breathing. She went to her nearest urgent care to find out what was making her so sick. Wendy began undergoing further respiratory distress and weakness while at the urgent care center.

Wendy was transferred to the nearest acute care hospital for intense medical workup and treatment. During examination, Wendy was found to have muscle weakness in her legs and arms. She was also noted to have decreased reflexes. She underwent a lumbar puncture and other neurological testing. She was found to have Guillain-Barré Syndrome (GBS), a rare nervous system disorder that results in nerve damage caused by the immune system's response to an infection or illness. During her acute stay, Wendy received intravenous immune globulin treatments along with OT, PT, SLP, and respiratory therapies.

Wendy's respiratory distress resolved and she did not need to undergo a tracheostomy. Her strength improved, but she was noted to have severe ataxia. After 5 days in acute care, Wendy transitioned to inpatient rehabilitation. She completed her comprehensive rehab program in two weeks with focus on safety and independence in her daily routine.

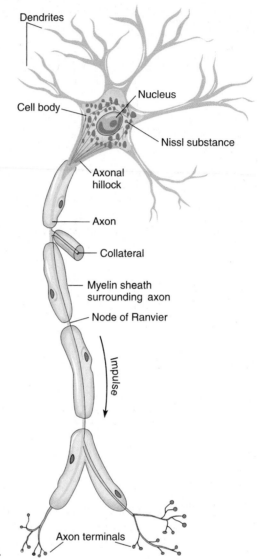

Anatomy of a multipolar neuron.

Source: Delmar/Cengage Learning.

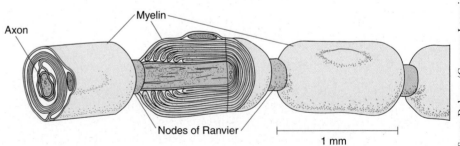

Anatomy of an axon of the peripheral nervous system lined with its myelin sheath.

Source: Delmar/Cengage Learning.

Wendy is a high-powered businesswoman and works full-time. She lives with her spouse and two teenage children (son, 14, and daughter, 16) in a rambler-style home. When not working, Wendy enjoys gardening and spending time with her family.

Wendy has completed inpatient rehabilitation and returned home safely, but she continues to have ongoing issues related to having GBS. She is transitioning to outpatient rehabilitation services where she will receive OT and PT. She no longer requires SLP services.

Analysis of Occupational Performance

Synthesis of Occupational Profile

Wendy is a 55-year-old left-handed woman who presents for outpatient OT secondary to ongoing problems with ataxia and decreased endurance because of GBS. Wendy and her inpatient practitioners believe that she will benefit from outpatient therapy services to address the occupations of return to work, home management, leisure, and driving.

Observed Performance in Desired Occupation/Activity

Activities of Daily Living

Wendy is not experiencing difficulties in her daily routine, except she needs to conserve her energy until she is cleared medically regarding potential recurrence of her GBS, typically at least 1-year post original diagnosis of the syndrome.

Functional Mobility: Wendy continues to be challenged by decreased coordination and ataxia when ambulating, so she is using a rolling walker and ambulating only short to moderate distances (i.e., 150 to 200 feet) at the time of the evaluation. Her endurance is poor, so she relies on a rental wheelchair for her long-distance mobility. Wendy needs increased time and at least 2 to 3 rest breaks when ambulating further than 200 feet. Furthermore, as she ambulates for longer distances, her ataxia increases and she has greater risk of falling. Although Wendy's work is willing to make accommodations for her, she needs to be ambulating longer distances (i.e., at least 300 to 500 feet) and using an assistive device less restrictive than a walker in order to have at least one hand free for performing parts of her essential job functions.

Leisure

Leisure Exploration: Wendy wants to explore options of how to get back to all of her gardening. She would like to either improve her skills regarding coordination or find ways to modify the tasks so that she does not have to ask for help from her spouse.

Leisure Participation: Wendy is an avid gardener. After discharge to home, she was able to get back to some of her gardening, but she has difficulty with deadheading and other tasks that involve increased dexterity. She also limits how much she kneels or bends down because her ataxia causes her to fall and she finds it challenging to get back up.

Social Participation

Family: Wendy's spouse is very supportive, but he works full-time. He is able to help around the house, but Wendy would love to return to all of her original occupations in their home. Wendy has two children who are teenagers. They do not drive and definitely feel the strain that Wendy cannot drive again yet.

Factors Influencing Performance Skills and Patterns

Motor Skills

Posture: Wendy's sitting balance has improved since she originally became ill. She is able to reach at least 2 to 3 feet out of her base of support including picking items up from the floor. She is able to accept moderate perturbations to her balance without loss of balance. Her static standing balance has also improved; however, when she moves in standing, she has moderate ataxia that gets in the way of doing everything. The ataxia also remains a safety concern, with increased falls when she ambulates greater than 200 feet or tries to reach a foot past her base of support.

Mobility: By the time of discharge from inpatient rehab, Wendy was able to ambulate 200 feet using a rolling walker with occasional safety concerns. Her ataxia puts her at greater risk for falling, but she has learned how to protect herself in case of a fall. She is able to get up from the floor with minimal physical assistance. Wendy needs to progress to using a cane or nothing in order to be able to complete occupations such as gardening and essential job functions at her work.

Coordination: Wendy's fine motor coordination is less impaired than her gross motor coordination, but as she fatigues, she has difficulty with detailed tasks such as writing and using the computer. Although the inpatient OT recommended that Wendy refrain from driving, she did try to drive in a vacant parking lot once with her spouse. She had difficulties switching between the brake and accelerator and would even miss the pedal sometimes. She tried to turn on the indicator for turning and would miss because of her ataxia. When making turns in the parking lot, Wendy would have difficulty keeping the turns smooth. She would also have difficulty turning in an acceptable turning radius.

Strength and Effort: Wendy becomes tired easily now that she has less structure at home compared to when she was in the hospital and had scheduled rest breaks in her daily inpatient rehabilitation schedule. However, her overall strength has improved compared to when she was first diagnosed with GBS.

Energy: Wendy feels as if she has more energy since her original illness. However, now that she is back home she finds that she forgets to schedule rest breaks and gets over-fatigued. She is worried about how low her energy remains. She is accustomed to keeping herself busy and is having difficulty limiting her activity level. Wendy wants to return to work, where she will need to maintain a certain energy level with her business clients (e.g., 30 to 60 minutes of continuous activity and communication without a break).

Process Skills

Knowledge: Wendy demonstrates keen understanding and awareness of her current limitations and goals for her continued reintegration back into her normal routine and responsibilities. She is highly involved in setting her outpatient rehabilitation goals and advocating for her ability to achieve her full potential.

Habits and Routines

Wendy has been able to get back into some of her usual habits and routines, although she has had to learn to incorporate energy-conservation techniques throughout her day. This need for rest breaks has forced Wendy to pay better attention to what she is doing and how she feels. As a result, Wendy would like to figure out a way to get back to doing many of her occupations more automatically.

Roles

Wendy has been able to resume many of her life roles, but she needs to continue to pace herself to avoid excessive fatigue. She desires to work toward return to her role as a businesswoman and regain independence with driving.

Factors Influencing Context(s)

Cultural

Wendy and her family have a strong Christian faith. She also has a strong work ethic and has found it difficult to be on medical leave of absence.

Physical

Wendy's work is eager for her return. They are willing to make any accommodations that are necessary. In spite of this, Wendy will need to ambulate long distances (i.e., between 300 to 500 feet) with a cane or no assistive device throughout her day. Once she is at her office, she will be able to sit as needed. Wendy does not have any other physical barriers to overcome or be modified.

Social

Wendy's spouse and children remain supportive. She has a strong network of friends who have proved supportive while she continues to regain energy at home.

Personal

Wendy prides herself in being a successful, independent businesswoman. She values her marriage and family responsibilities.

Synthesis of Abilities and Deficits

Facilitators to Occupational Performance

Wendy has made wonderful gains in resuming her basic daily routine. She demonstrates understanding and ability to apply the need to pace her activities to avoid recurrence of her illness. She is motivated to tackle her decreased coordination and ataxia so that she can return to performing more parts of her home management, driving, and work.

Barriers to Occupational Performance

Wendy is still at risk for recurrence of GBS, so she needs to pace herself. The fast pace of her job does not always fit with her need for energy conservation. Furthermore,

Wendy's ataxia and decreased coordination make it not only challenging but unsafe to return to driving, an occupation she needs to perform to get to her work site and to engage fully in her responsibilities as a mother in driving her teenagers to various school and extracurricular commitments.

Intervention

Intervention Plan

Collaborative Client Goals that are Objective and Measurable

Wendy would like to return to work, driving, and all aspects of gardening.

Wendy has an anticipated duration of treatment of 2-3 months with an estimated frequency of 2-3 treatment sessions per week. By the time of discharge, Wendy will perform the following:

1. Tasks related to return to work with good understanding of energy conservation techniques
2. Good understanding of driving screen recommendations
3. Increase reaction time by 0.5 seconds in applying brake or accelerator without overshooting
4. Increase activity tolerance to 30 minutes before needing a break in order to complete tasks related to work
5. Increase Berg Balance score to greater than 45 out of 56 to reduce fall risk during activities like gardening and cleaning
6. Cook a complex meal (entree and two side dishes) from an ambulatory level in less than 1 hour

Discharge Needs and Plan

Wendy needs to be able to improve her skills and determine modifications necessary for return to work, driving, and gardening. Depending on her performance on the driving screen, she may need to perform a behind-the-wheel evaluation. After intense outpatient rehabilitation, it is planned that Wendy will not need on-going OT other than the driving evaluation. However, she may benefit from annual check-ups with a physiatrist until she has fully recovered from her GBS.

Intervention Implementation

Therapeutic Use of Occupations and Activities

Occupation-Based Activities

Functional mobility

Driving

Gardening

Work

Cleaning

Cooking

Purposeful Activities

Practice various parts of office work
    organizing and filing paperwork
    composing and reading e-mail
    writing memos

Practice components of gardening

Practice complex meal preparation

Practice alternating between applying brakes and accelerator

Practice coordination for turning on indicator and turning steering wheel

Practice balance skills in varying tasks and environmental conditions

Preparatory Methods

Exercises

Transitional movements

Fine and gross motor coordination

Dynamic standing

Elicit musculoskeletal responses necessary for movement and balance

Consultation Process

Collaborate to determine the following:

    Best method for setting up work environment

    Best method and potential equipment for return to safe driving

    Potential modifications for improving participation in occupations such as gardening and complex meal preparation at home

    Methods on safety awareness and compensatory strategies for effective fall prevention

Education Process

Educate client in potential hazards with ataxia regarding return to safe driving

Intervention Review

Daily informal meetings set with OT to review progress, review treatment plan, and make modifications as needed.

Outcomes

Along with reviewing progress toward Wendy's objective goals, therapy will focus on her ability to resume participation in her role as a businesswoman and further expand her successful participation in her spouse and mother roles.

Questions

1. Complete an activity analysis of the occupation of driving.

2. Given your analysis, what are the specific component skills found in driving that need to be addressed with Wendy because of her ataxia and decreased coordination?

3. Describe a few treatment sessions that you would set up to accomplish return of these component skills for driving?

4. Describe the discussion you would have with Wendy regarding how you planned to accomplish her goals of return to work. What additional therapeutic activities might you give Wendy in order to increase the possibility of return to work?

5. Wendy confides that she is still practicing driving with her spouse in spite of her safety issues. What are your responsibilities as a professional?

6. In preparing to return to work, you have Wendy complete a weekly tracking tool regarding her activities throughout the week. She completes the schedule log for the week and brings it back to you for review. You analyze her patterns and find that at the beginning of the week, she is busy the entire day, and as the week progresses, she completes fewer activities. What are your recommendations?

7. You notice that Wendy is unsuccessfully trying to complete complex activities in the afternoon. You know from research that people should match the complexity of a task to their fatigue level. Furthermore, research shows that thought processes are clearer from 8 a.m. to 12 p.m. and from 6 p.m. to 8 p.m.; how would you instruct Wendy to adjust her weekly activities?

8. After being discharged from outpatient therapy services, Wendy completes the behind-the-wheel evaluation for driving with an OT certified in driving. During the evaluation, she is found to have continued difficulty with safely alternating quickly between the brake and accelerator. Her ability to turn has improved after therapy with you, but when distracted Wendy still has difficulty turning quickly and ends up in the wrong lane. She returns to you for continued outpatient services; what would you do?

Reference

Brain & Nervous Center Health Center. Guillain-Barré Syndrome Topic Overview. Retrieved off WebMD Medical Reference on August 2, 2008, from http://www.webmd.com/brain/tc/guillain-barre-syndrome-topic-overview

Florence

OUTPATIENT REHABILITATION: DRIVERS REHABILITATION

Level of Difficulty: Easy

Overview: Requires an understanding of driving and community mobility for an elderly person; specifically requires understanding of component skills necessary for return to safe driving and how to establish restrictions that allow for continued independence with driving

Engagement in Occupation to Support Participation in Context(s)

Performance in Areas of Occupation: Retiree and friend

Primary Impairments and Functional Deficits: Decreased reaction time, divided attention, visual processing

Context: Elderly woman who values independence of driving

Occupational Profile

Florence is an 87-year-old woman in relatively good state of health who presented to her primary care physician with concerns regarding her ability to drive. She reported that she has noticed that, as she ages, certain aspects of driving have become more challenging. Upon further interview and examination, Florence's doctor suspects that decreased balance, reaction time, and ability to handle new situations that are distracting may affect her ability to drive safely. The doctor recommends Florence pursue a driving screen including a behind-the-wheel evaluation with an OT with driver's certification.

Florence has remained fairly active in her community. She lives in a senior home where she is able to get all of her meals if she does not feel up to cooking for herself. Weekly she gets together with friends on the other side of town to work on a sewing project. She also keeps active by playing bridge and bingo with people in her senior home. Florence still drives to go to doctor's appointments and to run such errands as grocery shopping.

Florence is being seen for outpatient OT to address return to driving. Based on findings, she will also participate in an outpatient behind-the-wheel evaluation around her senior home and on the nearest highway.

Observed Performance in Desired Occupation/Activity

Instrumental Activities of Daily Living

Community Mobility: Currently, Florence and her friends have been having concerns about her ability to drive. At the recommendation of her doctor, Florence was encouraged to participate in evaluation of her current abilities related to driving. She continues to drive, but she is interested in finding out areas in which she can improve and whether a trained practitioner has any suggestions about maintaining as much independence as possible in the community, especially because she does not have family in the area and has limited support for community mobility. She wants to be safe, but she does not want to find out that she can no longer drive, because it will be incredibly isolating.

The outpatient OT performs a series of evaluations to determine Florence's cognitive, physical, and emotional function related to driving. Here are the findings from the pre-driving screen. Note that results from the screen are only to provide an indication regarding safety with driving, while the most accurate results regarding ability to return to driving would be from a behind-the-wheel evaluation on the road by a practitioner with driving specialty certification.

Clinical Results in Preparation for Behind-the-Wheel Testing

Currently driving?   *Not in the last month.*

Restrictions?   *None.*

Any accidents in the last 3 years?   *None.*

Evidence of seizures?   *No.*

Medications?   *None.*

Pre-Vehicle Assessment				
Physical Skills	**Right Upper Extremity**	**Left Upper Extremity**	**Right Lower Extremity**	**Left Lower Extremity**
Strength	within functional limits	within functional limits	within functional limits	within functional limits
Coordination	within functional limits	within functional limits	below functional limits	within functional limits
Range of Motion	within functional limits	within functional limits	within functional limits	within functional limits
Sensation/ Proprioception	within functional limits	within functional limits	within functional limits	within functional limits

(Continues)

Pre-Vehicle Assessment *(Continued)*		
	Within Functional Limits	**Below Functional Limits**
Neck Rotation	✔	
Sitting Balance	✔	
Standing Balance		✔
Endurance	✔	
Wheelchair Mobility (manual or power)	Not Applicable	
Ambulation	Florence is able to ambulate moderate to long distances using a rolling walker. She has a risk for falls as noted by a score below 40 on the Berg Balance Test.	
Transfers	Florence is able to perform transfers with modified independence with increased time, need for equipment, and occasional safety concerns.	
Visual Skills	**Yes**	**No**
Glasses/ Contacts	✔	
	Within Functional Limits	**Below Functional Limits**
Visual Field (peripheral)	130 ✔	
Acuity	left eye 20/40 right eye 20/40 both eyes 20/40 ✔	
Color Discrimination	✔	
Traffic Sign Recognition (x/12 Correct)	10/12 ✔	
Stereopsis/ Depth Perception		✔
Contrast Sensitivity	✔	
Cognitive/ Perceptual Skills	**Within Functional Limits**	**Below Functional Limits**
Visual Processing Speed		✔
Visual Memory	✔	

(Continues)

Pre-Vehicle Assessment *(Continued)*			
Short Blessed Test (dementia screen); Score of 8 or above indicates dementia	✔		
Symbol Digit Score of 25 or less indicates concerns with driving			✔ 20
Weintraub Structured Array	✔ **Organized with 1 error; needed visual demonstration at beginning**		
Dynavision			
	Mode A	35	Score of 52+ considered safe driver
	Mode B	20	Score of 42+ considered safe driver
	Divided Attention	**20, but aware of all numbers**	Score of 35+ considered safe driver
	Continuous (4 minute)	150	Score of 200+ considered safe driver
	Within Functional Limits		**Below Functional Limits**
Ability to Follow Instructions	✔		
Insight	✔		
Useful Field of View			
	Crash Risk	**3 Moderate Risk**	
	Central Vision/ Processing Speed	**Some Difficulty**	
	Divided Attention	**Some Difficulty**	
	Selective Attention	**Normal**	

(Continues)

Pre-Vehicle Assessment *(Continued)*			
Hearing	Intact	Impaired	
Hearing Aids	**Yes;** they still do not improve clarity adequately	No	
Driving Simulator	Florence was able to put on her seat belt, adjust the seat, and start the car with increased time. She was able to apply both the accelerator and brake, but she needed increased time to do so especially when needing to stop or start suddenly. She was able to turn the steering wheel with increased time, but she had difficulties navigating left-hand turns. She was consistently able to follow directions from the trainer on the simulator as long as the volume was turned up and background noises were kept to a minimum. She preferred to drive just below the speed limit and appeared to have difficulty if there was too much traffic. She was able to wait for pedestrians safely although she needs to use her mirrors better to check for blind spots.		

In-Vehicle Assessment Pre-Road Performance		
	Within Functional Limits	**Below Functional Limits**
Unlock/Lock Doors	✔	
Entry/Exit of Vehicle	✔	
Adjustment of Seat	✔	
Adjustment of Mirrors	✔	
Seat Belt Use	✔	
Operation of Accelerator/Brake	✔	
Reaction Time of Gas to Brake		✔
Operation of Steering	✔	
Operation of Secondary Controls		✔

Type of vehicle used   **Sedan**   Mini-Van   Full Size Van   Other
Seating   **Regular**   Wheelchair   Torso Support   Extra Cushions   Other
Adaptive Equipment Used: **None**
Mechanical Hand Control (type:)
Steering Device (type:)
Left Foot Accelerator
Gas/Brake Block

Right-Hand Turn Signal
Modified Secondary Controls (specify:)
Other: (specify:)

On-the-Road Performance			
Vehicle Operation		**Within Functional Limits**	**Below Functional Limits**
	Acceleration/ Braking		✔ at higher speeds
	Steering/Vehicle Tracking	✔	
	Right Turns	✔	
	Left Turns		✔
	Parking and Backing Maneuvers	✔	
Traffic Flow		**Within Functional Limits**	**Below Functional Limits**
	Speed Adjustment		✔ maintains speed limit, but difficulty with adjustment at higher speeds
	Lane Changing/ Merging	✔	
	Vehicle Spacing, Following Distance	✔	
	Positioning/Speed for Stopping	✔	
	Techniques/ Procedures at Intersections		✔
Scanning and Observation Techniques		**Within Functional Limits**	**Below Functional Limits**
	Use of Mirrors	✔	
	Checking Blind Spots		✔
	Identification/ Compliance with Signs	✔	
	Dynamic Scanning of Environment		✔ at higher speeds or with increased traffic
	Uncontrolled Intersections		✔

(Continues)

On-the-Road Performance *(Continued)*			
Concentration/ Attention to Driving Task		**Within Functional Limits**	**Below Functional Limits**
	Managing Distractions		✔
	Accommodating to Unpredictable Change		✔
	Anticipation/ Planning in Traffic	✔	
	Sustained Attention	✔	
	Attending to Multiple Stimuli	✔ **at slower speeds with limited traffic**	✔ **at higher speeds or with increased traffic**
		Within Functional Limits	**Below Functional Limits**
Perceived Risk		✔	
Path Finding Skills		✔ **for familiar locations**	✔ **for new locations**
Knowledge of Traffic Rules		✔	
Judgment/ Decision Making		✔	
Emotional Response		✔	
Freeway/ Highway Driving		**Within Functional Limits**	**Below Functional Limits**
	Entering/Exiting		✔
	Lane Changing/ Merging		✔
	Speed Adjustment		✔
	Positioning/ Spacing		✔
	Awareness of Traffic		✔

Recommendations/ Summary

This client demonstrates potential to safely operate a motor vehicle with restrictions.

Synthesis of Abilities and Deficits

Facilitators to Occupational Performance

Florence is aware that as she has gotten older, her balance and reaction time have also changed. She demonstrates good insight and judgment into wanting to find a way to resume driving safely so that she can get around in her familiar environment during the day.

Barriers to Occupational Performance

Florence demonstrates decreased reaction time, divided attention, ability to manage multiple distractions, hearing, ability to handle higher levels of traffic and speed, which are affecting her ability to resume driving in less familiar or high-traffic areas especially on the freeway. She has a limited support system in the area and does not want to ask her friends to take her places because of perceiving that she will be too much of a burden on them.

Intervention Implementation

Therapeutic Use of Occupations and Activities

Occupation-Based Activities

Community

Mobility

Driving

Alternative transportation

Purposeful Activities

Reaction time

Divided attention

Managing a task with distractions

Consultation Process

Collaborate to determine alternative transportation for successful community mobility

Education Process

Provide education regarding results of on-the-road driving evaluation and recommendations regarding driving including potential restrictions

Intervention Review

Daily informal meetings set with occupational therapist to review progress, review treatment plan, and make modifications as needed.

Outcomes

Florence has an anticipated duration of treatment 2 weeks, with an estimated frequency of 1 to 2 treatment sessions. By the time of discharge, Florence will demonstrate the following:

1. Good understanding of recommendations regarding return to driving

2. Identify 3–4 strategies for resuming safe driving and successful participation in community mobility with restrictions found during driver evaluation

3. Good understanding of home exercise program to work on increasing areas related to component skills of driving

Questions

1. Write a more comprehensive summary/recommendations section for Florence and her primary care physician based on the findings from the pre-vehicle assessment, in-vehicle assessment, and on-the-road performance.

2. Create a home program for Florence with focus on increasing reaction time and ability to handle multiple stimuli. What other component skills do you think that Florence will need to improve to increase her chance of successful return to driving in familiar areas? What additional exercises would you add to her home program to address these skills?

3. You and the OT determine that Florence would benefit from a few sessions of training behind the wheel. Describe how you would set up the session to help reinforce the restrictions recommended along with providing an opportunity for Florence to practice driving in a controlled setting.

4. What are your ethical and legal responsibilities regarding reporting any concerns related to Florence's driving?

5. Part of Florence's restrictions is that she should no longer drive at night. Unfortunately, Florence has a weekly sewing group that she attends devotedly. She thrives on keeping her hands and mind active and loves maintaining connections with long-time friends in the group. Florence consults you for advice. What would you say and what might you add to the treatment session to help her get to her meeting safely?

6. What are some additional resources or recommendations that might be helpful to Florence in getting her to doctor's appointments or the grocery store?

Anupam

OUTPATIENT REHABILITATION

Level of Difficulty: Moderate

Overview: Requires an understanding of stroke rehabilitation in a traditional outpatient setting (specifically an understanding of higher-level cognitive retraining and neuro-reeducation of the upper extremity), and an understanding of the cultural and personal issues of a new mother from India

Engagement in Occupation to Support Participation in Context(s)

Performance in Areas of Occupation: Spouse, computer software programming consultant, and new mother

Primary Impairments and Functional Deficits: Decreased right upper extremity strength and function, shoulder pain, headaches, fatigue, decreased higher-level cognition, ongoing decreased understanding regarding effect of personal factors and stroke

Context: New mother who was primary breadwinner of Indian family

Occupational Profile

Anupam is a 30-year-old right-handed married woman from India who sustained a stroke after the birth of her son. She was hospitalized and treated in acute care for 3 days for complete workup and medical management of her stroke. Once stabilized, Anupam transitioned to inpatient rehabilitation for 3 weeks.

Anupam is a new mother of a 4-week-old son. She is married and lives in a house with multiple steps both outside and inside. Before her stroke, Anupam worked full-time as a computer programmer/consultant. She was the primary breadwinner for herself and her spouse. She and her spouse value the worker role, while parenting is seen to be a role of the extended family.

While in inpatient rehabilitation for 3 weeks, she was able to improve her basic daily routine to an independent level, but she had residual problems with higher-level cognition and 1/5 to 2/5 muscle strength in her right upper extremity. Furthermore, she is now experiencing pain in her right upper extremity. Anupam presents to outpatient rehabilitation to work on skills necessary for resuming occupations such as return to driving, return to work, mother role, and spouse role.

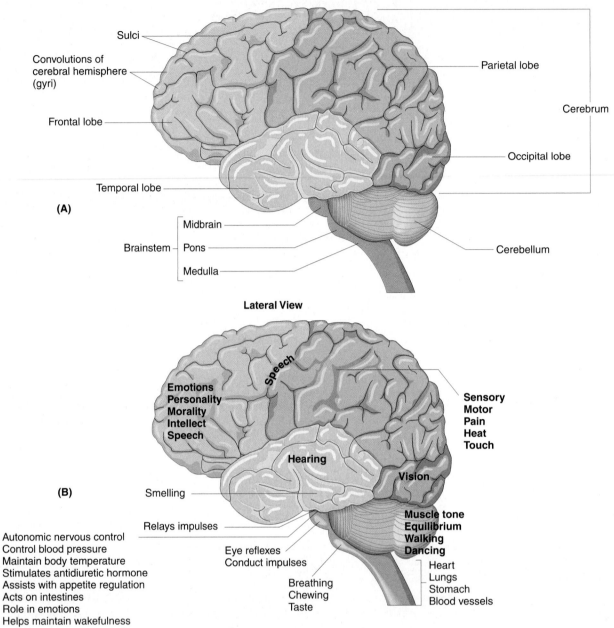

Source: Delmar/Cengage Learning.

A. The parts of the brain. B. Areas of brain function.

Analysis of Occupational Performance

Synthesis of Occupational Profile

Anupam is a 30-year-old female who sustained a stroke resulting in right hemiparesis and cognitive deficits after the birth of her son. She has completed acute and inpatient rehabilitation and is now being seen by outpatient OT to work on skills for resuming driving, return to work, and her life roles of mother and spouse.

Observed Performance in Desired Occupation/Activity

Activities of Daily Living

Bathing: Anupam is able to bathe independently with increased time and equipment. She remains seated in the shower for safety and increased ability to wash her feet, but she is unable to use right arm to assist with any part of the task of bathing.

Dressing: Anupam is able to perform total body dressing with increased time, occasional safety concerns, and adaptive equipment. She is able to use hemi-techniques to get dressed with increased time. She demonstrates occasional safety concerns especially with lower dressing and requires increased time. Anupam uses a buttonhook to manage buttons and zippers in her clothing.

Functional Mobility: Anupam is able to perform all aspects of bed mobility independently with increased time and good safety awareness. When ambulating, Anupam demonstrates occasional safety concerns related to dynamic balance and occasionally demonstrates decreased right-sided attention. She is able to ambulate long distances (over 500 feet) without an assistive device, but she reports ongoing issues with fatigue and limited endurance.

Toileting Anupam is able to toilet herself independently. She uses a buttonhook for fasteners. She does not need any equipment on her toilet and can get on and off a standard toilet seat with increased time.

Instrumental Activities of Daily Living

Child Rearing: Anupam is a new mother of a 4-week-old son. She is having difficulty with changing his diaper with one hand, bathing him, and carrying him. Since returning home from the hospital, Anupam is trying to breastfeed her son, but she is having difficulty with achieving a successful position because of her right-sided hemiparesis. Anupam's spouse has been taking over primary caregiving responsibilities. They have discussed the possibility of taking her son to India so that he can be taken care of by Anupam's parents while she focuses on recovering from her stroke.

Community Mobility: For community ambulation, Anupam requires supervision because of higher-level cognitive deficits and increased risk of falls because of decreased dynamic balance and fatigue. When ambulating outside, Anupam can become distracted and demonstrates increased safety concerns resulting in a need for supervision by her spouse.

Before her stroke, Anupam drove. She is not driving currently, but she is eager to participate in evaluation and treatment related to return to driving. While in inpatient rehabilitation, she was noted to have difficulties with right-sided control of the steering wheel, brake, and accelerator. She also demonstrated delayed processing time, slow reaction time, difficulty with divided attention, difficulty with endurance, and decreased attention/concentration.

Financial Management: Before her stroke, Anupam was responsible for the household financial management. While in inpatient rehabilitation she had difficulties with simulated finances, including balancing the budget, organization, attention to detail, attention/concentration, and error identification. It was recommended that Anupam's spouse take over the family's finances for now. Anupam would like to work on skills necessary to resume her occupation of financial management for her household.

Health Management and Maintenance: Upon discharge from inpatient rehabilitation, Anupam was requiring supervision regarding medication management. Her spouse helps to set up her medications for the week and then reminds her to take them throughout the day. Anupam requires assistance to call and set up medical appointments. She has difficulty recalling when appointments are so her spouse not only reminds her, but he also takes her to all appointments. Anupam continues to demonstrate decreased understanding regarding how to incorporate healthier food choices and cooking for lowering hypertension and cholesterolemia, two of her risk factors for recurrence of a stroke.

Home Establishment and Management & Meal Preparation and Cleanup: Anupam requires minimal assistance for performance of occupations in home management, meal preparation, and cleanup. Anupam's spouse has been cooking since her return home from the hospital. Anupam is able to help with cooking but is challenged by her inability to use her right upper extremity. She demonstrates difficulty with planning out menus that account for low sodium and cholesterol. She has difficulty with organizing all parts of cooking, especially when trying to complete multiple steps or components of a meal. She needs cues for dividing her attention between items when cooking more than one thing for a meal. When distracted by something such as a ringing telephone, Anupam demonstrates increased difficulty in preparing a meal.

Shopping: Anupam has not attempted to go shopping with her spouse or by herself because of her inability to drive. While she was in inpatient rehabilitation, she participated in a community outing to the mall, where she had difficulties with fatigue, path finding, distractibility, and money management.

Education

Formal Educational Participation: Anupam completed graduate training in India for computer programming with high honors.

Work

Job Performance: Anupam worked full-time as a computer programmer/consultant. She has been unable to return to work since her stroke and is on temporary disability. She and her spouse value the worker role and she was the primary moneymaker for their family. Her position required constant cognitive demands, especially regarding time management, divided attention, prioritization, problem solving, organization, and attention to detail. She was responsible for communicating about projects to clients on the phone and in person. She needed excellent typing skills and understanding of multiple computer programs and how to trouble shoot errors. Anupam is interested in returning to work and needs to have help in determining any accommodations that she might ask of her employer so that she can resume making money for her family.

Retirement Preparation and Adjustment: Anupam has planned for retirement in her 60s and has saved accordingly into a 401K and IRA. She is less well prepared for the potential of inability to return to work as a computer programmer/consultant.

Leisure

Leisure Participation: Because of their strong work ethic, Anupam and her spouse did not engage in any leisure activities.

Social Participation

Community: Anupam and her family are strongly connected with a small Indian community in her area. They are supportive of trying to help her to return to work and are willing to help in the role of parent to her newborn son, because Anupam's extended family still lives in India.

Family: As was stated previously, Anupam is a new mother of a 4-week-old son. Since her stroke, Anupam's spouse has assumed the primary caregiver role. They have discussed the possibility of their son being raised in India by extended family so that Anupam can focus on recovery from her stroke and more specifically return to work. Anupam's spouse is supportive through taking care of their son or arranging so that Anupam can return to driving and work. However, he is not incredibly emotionally supportive. He demonstrates decreased willingness and understanding of how Anupam's stroke has affected her cognitive function.

Peer, Friend: Anupam has a close network of friend's in the area that has been supportive by helping to provide meals and run errands. Her employer is also the spouse of a close friend.

Factors Influencing Performance Skills and Patterns

Motor Skills

Mobility: Anupam's static and dynamic balance are good, but when fatigued she loses her balance. She is able to reach 2 feet out of her base of support. She is able to maintain single-leg stance on the left leg for 15 seconds, but she is unable to maintain single-leg stance on the right leg without additional steadying support of her left upper extremity. She is able to ambulate long distances (i.e., over 500 feet) inside and outside without an assistive device, but is limited by fatigue, distractibility, and right-sided inattention.

Strength and Effort: Anupam demonstrates 5/5 strength on her left side, roughly 4/5 strength in her right lower extremity, and 1/5 to 2/5 strength in her right shoulder, 3/5 in her right elbow, and 3/5 in her right hand. When she tries to use her right upper extremity, she has pain in her shoulder that is distressing and rates it as 7 out of 10, with 10 being unbearable or excruciating pain.

Energy: Anupam reports issues with ongoing fatigue throughout her day. She needs frequent breaks (i.e., a 5-minute break every 30 minutes) and finds that everything takes her much longer to complete, even for her basic daily routine.

Process Skills

Knowledge: Although Anupam is able to understand basic information and communicate her needs; she has difficulty following more complicated conversations. She is easily distracted by interruptions. She needs increased time to process information and needs to write everything down so that she gets all of the necessary details. She continues to demonstrate decreased knowledge about the more permanent and long-lasting effects from her stroke.

Habits and Routines

Anupam has been able to resume some of her daily routine and habits for her basic routine. However, she is finding that routines and habits that were once effective are no longer successful, because of higher-level cognitive dysfunction and impaired personal factors (e.g., fatigue/pacing, arousal/attention, physical symptoms, and negative feelings about disposition) and situational factors (e.g., external environment distracters and multitask demands). She has difficulty engaging in habits fully and functionally because of ongoing deficits with executive function (e.g., the ability to initiate and stop actions, to monitor and change behavior as needed, to plan future behavior when faced with novel tasks or situations, and abstract reasoning), external distracters in her environment, and decreased ability to handle multitask demands.

Roles

Since returning home, Anupam has had difficulty participating in her new role as mother. She is limited in her ability to help with home management because of her higher-level cognitive issues, not to mention inability to use her right upper extremity functionally. Anupam and her spouse remain together, but they have issues with emotional supportiveness and sexual intimacy after her stroke. She is currently unable to participate in her work role as a computer programmer, which has proven to be a huge loss and strain because she was the primary breadwinner and her cultural background values the ability to be productive over all other life roles.

Factors Influencing Context(s)

Cultural

Anupam and her spouse have lived in the United States for the past 10 years. Although they have assumed some level of integration into American culture, Anupam maintains a strong involvement and adherence to Hindu religion and way of life, including fasting to remain connected to the Supreme Being.

Physical

Anupam is physically able to get around her home and in the community. However, she is unable to reach with her right arm to get things out of higher cabinets.

Social

As was stated before, Anupam and her family are strongly involved in the Hindu community in her area. Anupam and her spouse were married according to Hindu tradition, including following caste and partner selection by Anupam and her spouse's parents.

Personal

Anupam is a 30-year-old woman who is a new mother and prides herself in her ability to provide for her family as a computer programmer.

Synthesis of Abilities and Deficits

Facilitators to Occupational Performance

Anupam is aware of some of her cognitive and physical deficits that are barriers for return to work, driving, and parenting. She is motivated to work on whatever skills are necessary for her to return to work as a computer programmer. Anupam's spouse is willing to assume more responsibilities in their family so that Anupam can focus completely on regaining function.

Barriers to Occupational Performance

Although Anupam recognizes some deficits that remain from her stroke, she is less able to identify the higher-level cognitive deficits and fatigue that are affecting her ability to resume life habits, routines, and roles. She is limited by decreased right upper extremity function and pain in her shoulder. She has difficulty with fatigue and headaches. Anupam's spouse is neither emotionally supportive nor understanding of higher-level deficits that are affecting successful and realistic return to previous and new life roles. Anupam's Hindu culture is strong and sometimes conflicts with her current level of function and participation level in the community.

Intervention

Intervention Plan

Collaborative Client Goals that are Objective and Measurable

Anupam would like to return to driving and work. She would like to have more energy to be able to resume roles at home, including the family's financial management.

Anupam has an anticipated duration of treatment 6 to 12 months, with an estimated frequency of 1-hour treatment sessions twice weekly. By the time of discharge, Anupam will perform the following:

1. Establish and maintain consistent routine of completing activity prioritization checklist for the day/week/month with modified independence
2. Identify personal and situational factors and how to compensate for them to increase ability to establish successful habits and routines at home and in preparation for return to work
3. Identify 3–5 specific interruptions and how to minimize them during a simulated work routine with minimal cues
4. Demonstrate good understanding of recommendations regarding return to work including time management on projects, choice of familiar versus new projects, single- versus multiple-piece projects, etc.
5. Demonstrate good understanding of driving recommendations
6. Identify and increase parenting skills needed along with potential modifications to engage in mother role, at least as shared responsibility with spouse

Discharge Needs and Plan

Anupam would like to return to driving, return to work, and be a more active participant as a spouse and new mother of their newborn son. She needs to improve both physical and cognitive function to achieve increased participation at a community level. Depending on her performance on the driving screen, she will most likely need a behind-the-wheel evaluation. After intense outpatient rehabilitation, Anupam will need vocational rehabilitation. She will benefit from annual checkups with a physiatrist because of ongoing issues related to aging after a stroke and potential issues with longer-term disability.

Intervention Implementation

Therapeutic Use of Occupations and Activities

Occupation-Based Activities

Driving

Working

Parenting

Home management

Complex meal preparation and cleanup

Purposeful Activities

Practice changing infant's diapers

Practice different holding patterns for feeding infant

Complete daily activity log for the week

Complete checklist to prioritize day

Organize ingredient list for cooking meal with an entree and one side dish

Shop for ingredients for cooking meal with an entree and one side dish

Complete work-related task with periodic interruptions of phone or e-mail

Work on tasks to increase reaction time in order to return to driving

Practice tasks involving divided attention

Practice turning a steering wheel with spinner knob and left hand

Preparatory Methods

Biofeedback

Physical agent modalities
    Neuromuscular electrical stimulation
    Transcutaneous electrical nerve stimulator (TENS)
    Hot or cold packs

Neuromuscular re-education

Strengthening

Stretching

Kineseotaping

Cognitive retraining

Consultation Process

Collaborate to determine personal factors that are contributing to performance inefficiencies and how to control these factors.

Education Process

Provide education and recommendations for the following:

Return to driving

Modifications to work role or alternative work options if return to computer programming is not realistic

Teach coping strategies for dealing with situational factors regarding return to work

Intervention Review

Daily informal meetings set with OT to review progress, review treatment plan, and make modifications as needed.

Outcomes

Besides reviewing progress toward Anupam's objective goals, therapy will focus on her ability to resume participation in her roles as spouse, mother, and worker.

Questions

1. Anupam's spouse comes to therapy one day and is loud and aggressive. How would you de-escalate the situation?

2. Anupam undergoes neuropsychological testing and is found to have severe deficits in executive function, working memory, speed of processing, ability to come up with alternate solutions, and visual spatial skills. What areas would you anticipate focusing on in therapy to help her return to work as a computer programmer?

3. Given the same deficits as stated in question 2, what areas would you focus on for helping Anupam return to driving?

4. Anupam brings in her daily activity log for the week. You notice that she appears to be doing most activities at the beginning of the week but is doing less by the end of the week. What might be explanations for this change in activity pattern? What would you provide as education for prioritizing and spreading out her activities throughout the week?

5. Given Anupam's physical and cognitive deficits, what reasonable accommodations might you recommend to her employer for her successful return to work?

6. How would you address Anupam's Indian and more specifically Hindu culture?

7. Plan out your treatment session to address increased right upper extremity function.

8. You notice that Anupam is complaining of pain that is spreading throughout her affected right upper extremity. When her hand is touched, she withdraws quickly and complains of a burning pain. The skin on her arm, especially in her hand, is dry, thin, and shiny. Finally, when you compare her two arms, her right arm is warm to touch and appears slightly swollen. What are some tools that you could incorporate to prevent problems with Anupam further developing Complex Regional Pain Syndrome?

Reference

Medical Encyclopedia. Complex Regional Pain Syndrome. Retrieved August 10, 2008, from http://www.nlm.nih.gov/medlineplus/ency/article/007184.htm. Using the search engine Google and key terms "shoulder hand syndrome."

Brad

OUTPATIENT REHABILITATION: HAND THERAPY

Level of Difficulty: Moderate

Overview: Requires understanding of treatment of nerve injuries in an adult in an outpatient hand therapy setting

Engagement in Occupation to Support Participation in Context(s)

Performance in Areas of Occupation: Full-time quality assurance machine inspector, father, adult son, boyfriend, and pet owner

Primary Impairments and Functional Deficits: Decreased sensation, decreased strength, decreased coordination, pain, decreased understanding of nerve entrapment effect on function and prevention

Context: Blue-collar worker and single parent

Occupational Profile

Brad is a 45-year-old man who presented to his primary care physician with progressive weakness, pain, and sensory changes in his arms. He is unable to recall a specific traumatic event that coincides with the changes in function, but instead he reports that he has been noticing changes for more than a year. He says that opening and manipulating small objects has become more challenging. He sometimes loses his grip on things, especially if he is not looking at his hands. At the end of a long workday, he reports needing to take a long rest break and pain medication to stop his elbows from hurting.

Brad works full-time as a quality assurance inspector for a machine shop. He needs to travel to various locations to inspect equipment to make sure that it is functioning correctly along with inspecting final products before they can be distributed to clients.

When not working, Brad spends time with his teenage son, for whom he functions as a single parent. They spend lots of time working around the house on various projects, especially fixing and maintaining cars. Brad is the primary caregiver to two cats and one dog. He is having difficulties with ambulating his dog; sometimes he drops the leash because of numbness and weakness in his hands.

Brad reports that although he has a good relationship with his girlfriend, he has been experiencing difficulty with sexual intimacy as a result of the problems with his hands.

In his clinical findings the primary care physician suspects issues with peripheral nerves but finds no other medical complications. He is recommending that Brad be seen by outpatient hand therapy for complete workup and treatment. Because of the possibility that Brad's problems stem from his work as a quality assurance inspector for a machine shop, the physician has also filled out necessary worker's compensation paperwork. Subsequent to the physician's findings, Brad is being seen by hand therapy for evaluation and then having a few ongoing treatment sessions to determine the source of his problems and provide prevention strategies, especially recommendations for work-site modification.

Analysis of Occupational Performance

Synthesis of Occupational Profile

Brad is a 45-year-old man who presents with progressive changes to his hand function over the past year. He is a quality assurance inspector for a machine shop, father, boyfriend, adult son, and pet owner. He presents for outpatient hand therapy to address positioning, exercises, splinting, and work-site recommendations to enhance occupational performance and prevent further decline in function.

Observed Performance in Desired Occupation/Activity

Activities of Daily Living

Bathing: Brad is able to bathe himself with increased time, but because of decreased strength in his hands he does not feel that he is able to clean himself thoroughly.

Dressing: Brad is able to get dressed with increased time for putting on socks, tying his shoes, and fastening snaps/buttons/zippers.

Functional Mobility: Brad is able to get around without difficulties.

Personal Grooming: Brad is independent with the tasks of grooming. He has difficulty holding his comb and razor, but he is able to perform all parts of grooming with increased time.

Sexual Activity: Brad has noticed difficulties with sexual activity because of decreased feeling and strength in his hands. It takes him longer to achieve an orgasm when masturbating. He also has difficulties pleasing his girlfriend because of decreased coordination in his hands. Changes in his sexual activity have been wearing heavily on Brad.

Sleep/Rest: Brad's sleep is fairly good, but he does notice that he sometimes wakes up with a feeling of pins and needles in his hands and fingers. Frequently, he sleeps with his elbows bent and both hands under his head.

Toileting: Brad is able to toilet himself independently, but he takes longer to make sure that he has wiped himself thoroughly after a bowel movement. Brad has difficulty zipping and buttoning/snapping his pants and has thought about limiting his wearing of certain clothing, such as his favorite jeans.

Instrumental Activities of Daily Living

Care of Pets: Brad has two cats and one dog. Although he is the primary caregiver for his animals, he needs to get help from his son to open bags and containers of food. Sometimes when he is walking his dog, he loses grip on the leash and the dog gets away from him.

Child Rearing: Brad is the primary parent for his teenage son. Although Brad maintains pleasant contact with his former spouse, Brad's son has chosen to live with his dad during his high school years. Brad and his son have a great relationship and they enjoy spending time together. Recently it has been more challenging for Brad to teach his son how to perform auto maintenance because of the changes in his hands.

Community Mobility: Brad is able to ambulate long distances (i.e., greater than 500 feet) and gets around his community by driving. He is able to drive safely, but he notices that sometimes he has to concentrate closely on his hands to make sure that he does not lose grip of the steering wheel.

Health Management and Maintenance: Overall, Brad is able to manage his health well, except that he is having difficulty opening his pill containers and needs to ask for assistance from his son. Brad sees a primary care physician every 1 to 2 years. He has been avoiding going to the doctor about the changes in his hands because he is worried about what the doctor will find.

Home Establishment and Management; Meal Preparation and Cleanup: Brad and his son share responsibilities for home management and meal preparation. He is able to perform all tasks with increased time when dexterity is needed.

Education

Formal Educational Participation: Brad completed high school and a few semesters of college.

Work

Job Performance: Brad works as a quality assurance inspector for a machine company. His typical day consists of propping on his elbows while looking through a magnifying lens to inspect various tools and parts before they are used. After a long day of inspecting, Brad needs to take ibuprofen and rest his arms because they hurt so much.

Leisure

Leisure Participation: Brad enjoys tinkering with his cars including a classic car. He is finding this challenging because of the numbness, decreased strength, and decreased coordination in his hands. Brad also enjoys going to movies with his son and girlfriend.

Social Participation

Community: Brad does not leave much time for socializing in his community because of his work demands.

Family: Brad is the primary parent to his teenage son, with whom he has a good relationship. Brad's parents live nearby and he helps to make sure that his father's diabetes is managed adequately.

Peer, Friend: Brad keeps to himself and his family except for spending time with his girlfriend. His girlfriend is supportive both physically and emotionally. However, she has noticed changes in their intimacy since Brad has had more difficulty with his hand function.

Factors Influencing Performance Skills and Patterns

Motor Skills

Mobility: As was stated before, Brad does not have difficulty with his mobility.

Strength and Effort: Brad's strength is 5/5 for all muscle groups proximal to his elbows. His right side is weaker than his left at 3/5 for all remaining movements and 4-/5 for his left. He has difficulty straightening out his 4th and 5th fingers on both hands. When asked to move more quickly, he has difficulty with accurate finger opposition. When an upper limb neurodynamic test is completed, Brad demonstrates positive signs for both the median and ulnar nerves on his right side and has mild signs on his left side.

Energy: Brad's energy is fairly good, but he does find that he tires easily at his job, and the fatigue worsens as his elbows start hurting more. When in pain, he finds that he needs to take breaks every 30 minutes for at least 2 to 3 minutes at a time.

Process Skills

Knowledge: Brad is uncertain what is contributing to his decreased hand function and pain in his elbows.

Habits and Routines

As Brad's hands have gotten worse, he has had interruption in some of his typical routines such as leisure pursuits and spending time with his son teaching him how to fix cars. Other than this, Brad does not feel that his habits and routines have been disrupted too much by the pain, numbness, and decreased coordination in his hands.

Roles

Brad is still working full-time, but he is finding it challenging. He is able to maintain being an involved father, but he also finds that he cannot interact with his son to teach him things like fixing cars. Brad is having difficulty taking care of his animals without the assistance of his son to open food containers. Brad prides himself in being able to check in on his parents to make sure that his father is managing his diabetes well. Brad is involved with his girlfriend, but the changes in his hand function have caused some difficulty in their sexual activity.

Factors Influencing Context(s)

Cultural

Brad is a Native American Indian, but because of his choice to focus on his family and work he is not well-connected to the Indian community.

Physical

Brad has no physical barriers other than the fact that opening containers is more challenging for him.

Social

Brad is focused on his family, his girlfriend, and his work.

Personal

Brad is a 45-year-old blue-collar worker who is a single parent of a teenager.

Synthesis of Abilities and Deficits

Facilitators to Occupational Performance

Brad is motivated to learn what is going on with his hands. He is able to identify clearly areas where he is having difficulties. Brad's son is able to help him if necessary. Brad's employer is receptive to modifying his work routine so that he can still complete his responsibilities with less potential for further injury.

Barriers to Occupational Performance

Brad has delayed getting his arms checked out. He has had difficulty with feeling, strength, and coordination for more than a year. He demonstrates positive signs for ulnar and median nerve entrapment, with the right side worse than the left. Brad's work demands prolonged and awkward positioning of his arms to perform quality assurance inspection of equipment.

Intervention

Intervention Plan

Collaborative Client Goals that are Objective and Measurable

Brad would like to learn why his hands have been getting worse and find ways to increase his strength and coordination while decreasing pain in his hands.

Brad has an anticipated duration of treatment of 1 to 2 weeks with an estimated frequency of 2-3 sessions. By the time of discharge, Brad will demonstrate the following:

1. Good understanding of home exercise program to be completed daily
2. Good understanding of positioning recommendations while working and sleeping

3. Good understanding of purpose, wear, and care of nighttime splint including ability to don/doff splints independently

4. Good understanding of work-site modifications to perform essential job functions with less risk of repetitive strain and entrapment injuries

Discharge Needs and Plan

Brad needs to be able to function better at work with less ongoing trouble with his hands. He needs to be able to learn a home program to limit permanent nerve damage including exercises, positioning, and splint wear. It is anticipated that after discharge from outpatient hand therapy Brad may need a work-site evaluation, especially if his employer demonstrates inability to modify Brad's job sufficiently to prevent further overuse injuries.

Intervention Implementation

Therapeutic Use of Occupations and Activities

Occupation-Based Activities

Dressing (managing socks and fasteners)

Personal grooming (managing razor and comb)

Sexual activity

Sleep/rest

Care of pets

Child rearing

Health management and maintenance

Work

Leisure

Purposeful Activities

Fixing car

Opening containers and manipulating small objects like pills

Walking dog

Inspecting machinery

Preparatory Methods

Ultrasound

Ice

Neural flossing

Range of motion

Strengthening and stretching exercises

Positioning

Splint fabrication

Orthotic fit

Consultation Process

Collaborate to determine ways to accomplish essential job functions without risk of further nerve entrapment or overuse injuries

Education Process

Client training in the following:

Equipment/splint/orthotic recommendations

Positioning during sleep and daytime to prevent nerve compression or repetitive strain

Home program for strength, coordination, range of motion, and neural flossing

Intervention Review

Daily informal meetings set with OT to review progress, review treatment plan, and make modifications as needed.

Outcomes

Besides reviewing progress toward Brad's objective goals, therapy will focus on his ability to resume participation in his roles as father, quality assurance inspector, and pet owner.

Questions

1. What type of splint might you fabricate to prevent contractures especially of the 4th and 5th digits? Brad reports that he is not wearing the splints at night; what might be some reasons for his perceived non-adherence to your recommendations? How might you increase adherence?

2. What other pieces of equipment might help with prevention and allow Brad's elbows to rest in a straighter position? How will you help to make sure that Brad can put these orthoses on by himself to increase chance of adherence?

3. You find that Brad's median and ulnar nerves have been compromised most likely from prolonged propping on his elbows at work. Establish an exercise program to work on the areas controlled by these two nerve groups.

4. You have physical agent modalities certification and would like to try ultrasound to help with reducing pain in Brad's elbows. What would your settings and complete treatment plan be? Would there be any contraindications or areas of concern? If so, what would they be?

5. Write a letter of medical necessity to Brad's employer and worker's comp case worker that outlines what his current limitations are and recommendations for modifying his work site to prevent further injury.

6. What are some purposeful activities that you would incorporate into Brad's treatment to address his current limitations and provide opportunities for increased coordination and strength?

7. Draw out positioning recommendations for daytime and nighttime. How will you encourage decreased sustained bending at Brad's elbows and wrists?

Reference

Liebenson, Craig. (1996). *Rehabilitation of the Spine: A Practitioner's Manual.* Wolters Kluwer/Lippincott, Williams, and Wilkins. Baltimore, MD.

George

OUTPATIENT REHABILITATION

Level of Difficulty: Difficult

Overview: Requires understanding of treatment of an adult with a dual diagnosis of spinal cord injury and brain injury with limited support system in an outpatient setting

---

Engagement in Occupation to Support Participation in Context(s)

Performance in Areas of Occupation: Full-time employee, adult son, and father

Primary Impairments and Functional Deficits: Decreased strength, coordination, mobility, sensation, energy, higher-level cognition, medical instability (autonomic dysreflexia and orthostatic hypotension), decreased understanding of the effect of spinal cord injury

Context: Divorced adult Caucasian man

Occupational Profile

George is a 49-year-old right-handed man who sustained both spinal cord and mild brain injuries during a motorcycle crash. He was not helmeted and lost consciousness for at least 5 minutes (initial GCS of 11). His trauma resulted in C6 AIS A tetraplegia and moderate brain injury. Initially his cervical spine was surgically stabilized and then he was placed in a halo vest for 3 months. He also underwent a tracheostomy owing to respiratory complications from the injury. His acute care course was complicated by a pulmonary embolism (PE) and pneumonia. He was medically stabilized within a month in acute care, after which he transitioned to inpatient rehabilitation for 5 weeks. The focus there was on prevention of secondary complications of his spinal cord injury including respiratory management, verbal direction of his cares, education regarding spinal cord injury and brain injury, and cognitive retraining. By the time of discharge from inpatient rehabilitation, George was able to eat and groom with adaptive equipment after setup, and he was able to verbally direct his cares with increased time.

Because his family was unable to provide the level of physical assistance required, George temporarily went to an SNF for ongoing healing and management of his

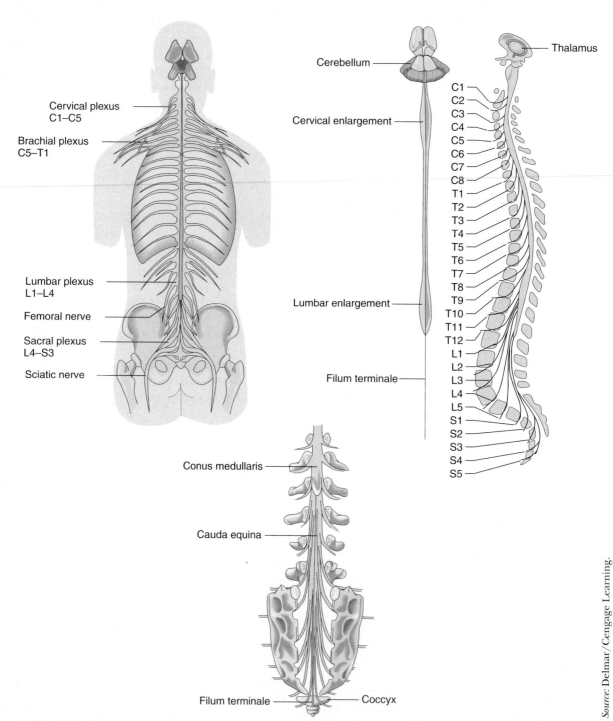

Spinal cord and nerves.

Source: Delmar/Cengage Learning.

halo vest. While at the SNF, he experienced complications of autonomic dysreflexia and development of sacral and ischial tuberosity pressure ulcers. Once his wounds healed and his halo vest was removed, he transitioned to a group home and received home health care, which focused on determining environmental modifications and establishment of a relationship with PCA services.

George continues to be challenged by decreased independence and social isolation. Overall, his cognitive deficits from his brain injury have resolved. He is being seen for initial evaluation and treatment in outpatient OT with focus on increased participation in his community and potential return to productive work. George's physiatrist has ordered PT, CM, TR, and psychology services in conjunction with outpatient OT.

Analysis of Occupational Performance

Synthesis of Occupational Profile

George is a 49-year-old right-handed man who sustained a traumatic SCI with now mild brain injury during a motorcycle crash 2 years ago. His rehabilitation course has been long and complicated. He has been seen throughout the rehabilitation continuum to address increased independence and verbal direction of his daily routine. George and his home health practitioners believe that he would benefit from outpatient therapy services to improve independence with bladder management, functional transfers (car, bed, toilet, shower), leisure participation, and knowledge of resources available for community participation after SCI.

Observed Performance in Desired Occupation/Activity

Activities of Daily Living

Bathing: George needs moderate assistance for bathing tasks. He now has a PCA to help him with his ADLs. He has learned to compensate for residual cognitive deficits of decreased memory and organization. He is able to instruct his PCA how to help him with bathing. George is able to help with washing the upper part of his body and the tops of his thighs, but he continues to need help to wash his back, bottom, front perianal area, calves, and feet.

Bowel and Bladder Management: Because of his C6 AIS A tetraplegia, George is unable to control his bowels or bladder without being on established bowel and bladder programs. He is on an every-other-day bowel program. He continues to require complete physical assistance to stimulate his bowels to move, in addition to occasional use of medications to prepare his bowels for evacuation. George is also on a successful bladder program and is catheterized intermittently every 6 hours. George has not learned how to perform self-catheterization. He is able to instruct his PCA in both his bowel and bladder programs. He is interested in determining whether he can learn to do his intermittent catheterization in order to have more independence and perhaps fewer hours of PCA services.

Dressing: Dressing tasks require George to get assistance with setup for upper body dressing and moderate assistance for lower body dressing. George is able to instruct his PCA in how to get him dressed and undressed. He is interested in learning how to dress himself.

Eating/Feeding: George is no longer on a modified diet and he is able to eat both with and without adaptive equipment. He requires increased time for tasks such as cutting up his food and opening containers.

Grooming: George requires more time and adaptive equipment to complete grooming tasks; he is therefore classified as modified independent. He is able to perform all parts of his grooming from a wheelchair level. The only adaptive equipment he needs to use for all of his grooming tasks is an adapted shaver and shaving cream can.

Functional Mobility: Overall, George's functional mobility has improved. He is able to roll from side to side with increased time. He requires moderate assistance to get from side lying into sitting up. He requires moderate assistance to lift his legs into bed, but can get them out with increased time. He requires moderate assistance for transfers across uneven surfaces (e.g., wheelchair to couch, wheelchair to standard toilet with a padded seat) and minimal assistance for transfers across level surfaces (bed to wheelchair, wheelchair to padded commode) using a lateral transfer with a transfer board. Occasionally, George has difficulty locking his elbows during transfers, which he needs to do to establish stability because of his upper extremity paresis and compromised trunk balance. He also has difficulty leaning far enough anterior and weight shifting in the direction opposite of the transfer. George would like to be able to transfer by himself so that he can get back into bed or get up without waiting for his PCA. He is able to get around by using a power wheelchair and can perform pressure relief and propulsion with increased time and use of the power tilt option. He is unable to manage the footrests and armrests of the wheelchair without assistance. George would like to try using a manual wheelchair to be able to get around in his group home better and to increase his overall strength and coordination. He would benefit from education about preservation of the upper limbs after spinal cord injury.

Sexual Activity: Since his injury, George has received resources and education about sexual dysfunction related to his SCI. His girlfriend Mary and he are no longer together because the permanence of George's disability and issues of her being a caregiver rather than partner became overwhelming. Before their breakup, Mary and George had been able to engage in sexual activity with the help of medication, equipment, and alternative positioning techniques.

Sleep/Rest: George no longer needs to be turned every 2 hours and he can roll side to side by himself if needed, therefore he is better able to sleep without interruptions. His sleep is also less disturbed by his bladder program because his PCA performs intermittent catheterization just before bed and right after he wakes up in the morning. His endurance is not as good as before his injury, but he is able to perform many of the tasks/occupations that he needs to in a given day with 2 to 3 rest breaks for every hour of activity.

Toilet Hygiene: George requires different levels of assistance for toilet hygiene depending upon where it is performed; he needs moderate assistance from the bed level and total assistance from the commode level. If George is back in bed, he is able to get his pants and underwear up and down for toileting. He is unable to wipe himself thoroughly from this level. He has not attempted to try toileting from a padded drop-arm commode.

Instrumental Activities of Daily Living

Community Mobility: George is now able to access public transportation or accessible medical vans for his community mobility. He occasionally gets rides from his parents and friends, but this is less frequent because it is difficult for others to transfer him in and out of their cars. Furthermore, most people do not have a way to transport George's power wheelchair, so he takes a loaner manual wheelchair that he is unable to propel. Because this makes him more dependent, he either chooses public transportation or limits how frequently he gets out of the group home. George's cognitive deficits are now subtler and he is able to compensate for them well. He is interested in pursuing return to driving, along with learning about accessible vehicle options/resources.

Health Management and Maintenance: George now goes to not only his primary physician, but also his physiatrist annually to help with medical management of his spinal cord and brain injuries. He is on fewer medications compared to when he was in the inpatient hospital, but he continues to need medications to help with management of blood pressure (was previously hypertensive and is now hypotensive) and diabetes mellitus (DM). He is able to recall all of his medications and when to take them, but he is having difficulty opening containers or holding the small tablets. Because of this, his PCA or a staff member in the group home helps him with medication management.

Home Establishment and Management: He needs total assistance for tasks related to home management. George would like to learn how to do light home management now that he is more settled in his group home.

Meal Preparation and Cleanup: Meal preparation and cleanup require maximal assistance. George can help with meal prep at the group home by cutting up vegetables or making sandwiches. He needs to be able to help with cooking a hot meal because this is one of the responsibilities at the group home.

Education

Formal Educational Participation: George graduated from college with a major in biology.

Work

Employment Interests and Pursuits: Before his injury, George was working full-time as a research technician in a biochemistry lab. His work demands involved frequent use of fine motor control, light lifting, and frequent communication. George has been unable to return to this work so he is currently on Social Security disability and welfare assistance. He would like to determine options for retraining through vocational services.

Leisure

Leisure Exploration While George was in inpatient rehabilitation, he met twice per week with the therapeutic recreation specialist to learn about leisure options available to him after a spinal cord injury. He also learned additional tips related to time management. George learned how to play cribbage with built-up pegs and a cardholder. Since he had a halo while he was an inpatient, he could not take advantage of the therapeutic pool. Now that his halo is removed, George would love to get into the pool to see how he moves and reestablish a means of exercise for his general well being. He remains interested in learning about all of his options and resources.

Leisure Participation: George still enjoys gardening, golfing, and riding motorcycles, but he has not participated in any of these leisure activities since his injury. Although he knows a little more about what is available to him as leisure resources, he is uncertain what parts of his leisure he can participate in or what other options are available to him.

Social Participation

Family: George's parents are still alive, but they live in a different town. They are older and, although emotionally supportive, they cannot provide physical support to George upon discharge. George still remains in contact with his ex-wife, in particular regarding decisions about their son Matthew. George shares custody of Matthew, and before his crash they would spend weekends together. Since his accident, George has gone on limited outings. He would like to plan a day trip to take with Matthew, even if it involved having his ex-wife come along to help. Because of the emotional strains and permanence of George's disability, he and his girlfriend have broken up. They remain friendly, but George does not see her frequently.

Peer, Friend: Although George had many friends before his crash he has become more isolated and is showing some signs of depression. He does not go out very much because he has to ask his friends to help with transfers. If he leaves the group home for long, he also has to ask someone to catheterize him. As a result, George does not keep in contact with many of his friends, except for a few who remain close.

Factors Influencing Performance Skills and Patterns

Motor Skills

Posture: George's balance has improved, although it is still not what it was before his injury. He can sit up in both a power and a manual wheelchair if there is a higher back to support him. He used to need a chest strap, but now needs it only when riding in a van. He no longer gets dizzy when sitting upright. He is able to maintain his balance on the side of the bed in short sitting for over a minute with supervision. He can sit up in bed with his arms behind him or holding onto his knees for support, but his posture is characterized by a posterior pelvic tilt.

Mobility: George remains unable to stand or ambulate. He has heard of the health benefits of a standing program after SCI. Now that the halo vest is off, he would like to be evaluated and trained for a program. George is able to get around with a power wheelchair with tilt control for independent pressure relief. He is able to propel the chair using a goal post joystick on his right side. He has a manual wheelchair that he uses for going out of the group home with friends and family, but he needs lots of help to propel the chair. He doesn't know the most efficient way to use his arms to push, and he needs to learn how to do so without causing any repetitive trauma to his shoulders.

Coordination: George is right-handed. Because of his injury, he has poor gross motor coordination and decreased fine motor coordination. Using the strength of his wrist extensors and tightness in his finger flexors, George has been able to pick up light objects such as 1-inch blocks and cotton balls using a tenodesis grasp. He is unable to pick up such things as his catheter or a piece of paper. He was measured and fitted for a metal tenodesis splint for his right hand by an orthotist while he was in home health care. He has not started training with the orthosis.

Strength and Effort: George's muscle strength is as follows: shoulder flexion 5/5, shoulder abduction 5/5, shoulder extension 5/5, elbow flexion 5/5, elbow extension 1/5, supination 4-/5, pronation 0/5, wrist flexion trace/5, wrist extension 4+/5, finger flexion 0/5, finger extension 0/5. Other than the elbow extension and wrist flexion movement noted above, George does not have movement below his level of injury.

Energy: George's endurance has been improving, but it continues to limit his ability to function fully in his daily routine. However, he is able to tolerate 1 hour of moderate activity with only 2 or 3 rest breaks.

Process Skills

George sustained trauma to his brain in addition to his spinal cord injury during his crash. Initially, he was having difficulty with attention (select, alternating, and divided), memory, organization, sequencing, functional problem solving, and error identification. While he was an inpatient, he learned a variety of strategies to help improve his cognitive function. Now he has higher-level residual deficits, specifically related to alternating and divided attention, organization, and complex functional problem solving.

Communication/Interaction Skills

George is able to communicate complex information with increased time. He is better able to follow conversations and communicate his thoughts 100% of the time even with distractions now, except when he is tired. While he was in inpatient rehabilitation, George learned how to write using a Wanchik's writer with a felt-tip pen because it requires less force to work than a ballpoint pen. George has also started training his voice to the voice-activated ECUs to operate lights, phone, television, and computer at his group home.

Habits and Routines

George's daily routines have become more automatic. He gets up early with the help of his PCA to perform his bowel program, shower, and get dressed. He is able to recall the timing of his medications and bladder management needs without cues. He has returned to a habit of having a morning cup of coffee while reading the newspaper which he turns using a page turner.

Roles

Initially, George was having difficulties in his roles as son, father, worker, and boyfriend because of physical and cognitive limitations. He has returned to being as involved with his son as possible, but he remains limited because of the difficulty of going on outings. George is physically unable to engage in his former worker role, which saddens him. He would like to learn about retraining or education opportunities so that he could get back to working. George is able to maintain his role as son to his parents and talks to them regularly on the phone. George and his girlfriend

Mary are neither intimately involved nor dating. Although he understands the reasons for their breakup, George is grieving the loss of his role as boyfriend.

Factors Influencing Context(s)

Cultural

George is Caucasian. He values his family, especially his son. George used to pride himself in his ability to work and is having difficulty with his inability to resume his work as a lab technician in the biochemistry lab.

Physical

George is living in a group home with four other housemates. The home is wheelchair accessible. There is a roll-in shower with necessary equipment for his showering. One of George's main physical limitations is his decreased community mobility secondary to lack of access to an accessible van and reliance on friends, family, or public transportation to get around. George is hesitant to go to new places or travel because of the uncertainty of accessibility.

Social

George's parents are still alive, but because of their own health conditions and ages they are not able to provide much physical assistance. George is divorced, but he stays in contact with his ex-wife and their son. George's ex-spouse has been supportive, trying to ensure that George remains connected with their son. George and Mary are no longer together, so he is missing that original social support. George has been isolating himself from his friends because he does not want to be a burden, but a couple of them remain supportive as much as their busy lives will permit.

Personal

George is a 49-year-old working right-handed divorced single man.

Synthesis of Abilities and Deficits

Facilitators to Occupational Performance

George remains motivated to get stronger and learn how to do more parts of his daily routine. His initial cognitive deficits have resolved and he has developed successful strategies to overcome residual deficits. His parents, ex-wife, and son provide strong emotional support. George's ex-wife is willing to help make it possible for George to plan and complete outings with their son so that he can remain connected as an involved father. George is able to pick up various light objects and his trunk control has improved since his original injury. George lives in an accessible group home and has a great relationship with his PCA. George is able to identify clear areas that he wants to focus upon during his outpatient episode.

Barriers to Occupational Performance

Although George's family remains emotionally supportive; they have limited ability to help with physical assistance or to provide 24-hour supervision. Although George's cognitive deficits have improved, he continues to have issues with higher-level deficits. His SCI remains complete and so his ability to perform all of his occupations without some level of assistance is challenging if not impossible.

Intervention

Intervention Plan

Collaborative Client Goals that are Objective and Measurable

George would like to get back into golfing, learn how to straight catheterize himself, and perform at least parts of his bowel program himself to increase his independence and reduce PCA service hours. George has an anticipated duration of treatment 1 to 2 years, with an estimated frequency of 60-minute sessions 2 to 3 times per week. By the time of discharge, George will perform the following:

1. Have triceps strength 2/5 to allow level lateral transfers with a transfer board independently

2. Have elbow extension to 180 degrees to allow elbows to extend during long and short sitting skills needed for lower body dressing and functional transfer tasks

3. Manipulate materials needed to complete self-catheterization independently using a tenodesis orthosis and possibly catheter inserter

4. Have shoulder depression and adduction strength of 4+/5 to allow increased independence with pressure relief in a manual wheelchair, clearance of his ischial tuberosities during transfers, and lower body dressing from a wheelchair or toilet level

5. Carry out upper body dressing independently

6. Have a good understanding of resources and adaptations needed for return to golfing as evidenced by participating in golfing at least twice

7. Have a good understanding of resources for accessible vehicles and steps necessary to pursue return to driving as evidenced by completing driving screen and setting an appointment for a behind-the-wheel driving evaluation

Discharge Needs and Plan

George needs to be able to have more opportunities for increased independence and participation at a community level. He needs to work on strengthening, stretching, adaptive equipment training, and PCA training. Because of ongoing issues with his mood and the challenges with his disability and increasing isolation, he will benefit from referral to psychology services. At discharge, he will benefit from ongoing referral to vocational services and a behind-the-wheel driving evaluation that includes addressing training for adapted driving controls.

Intervention Implementation

Therapeutic Use of Occupations and Activities

Occupation-Based Activities

Upper body dressing

Functional transfers

Self-catheterization

Toileting

Bowel management

Leisure exploration and participation
    Golfing
    Swimming
    Gardening

Driving

Health maintenance
    Medication management

Purposeful Activities

Practice identifying and picking up materials for self-catheterization

Practice using an adapted putter

Water flowers using adapted hose and watering can

Reach for sock or shoe while in long sitting

Practice putting on and taking off a shirt

Practice rolling side to side to lower pants in preparation for bowel program

Practice opening various medication containers and setting up medications for the week

Practice reaching for digital stimulation while seated on padded drop-arm commode

Preparatory Methods

Biofeedback and neuromuscular electrical stimulation (NMES) to both triceps

Fitting and training for tenodesis orthosis

Fine and gross motor coordination

Stretching and strengthening programs

Short and long sitting

Consultation Process

Collaborate to determine the following:

    Best equipment needs for self-catheterization and bowel management

    Best adaptations and technique for return to golfing and swimming

    Best adaptation for improved participation in self-medication

Education Process

PCA training about assistance and supervision needs and optimal facilitation of George's participation

Education about spinal cord injury (bowel, bladder, skin, pressure relief, equipment needs, neuroanatomy of injury, orthostatic hypotension, autonomic dysreflexia, and sexual function)

Education and resources related to return to driving and accessible vehicle options

Intervention Review

Daily informal meetings set with OT to review progress, review treatment plan, and make modifications as needed.

Outcomes

Along with reviewing progress toward George's objective goals, therapy will focus on his ability to resume participation in his roles of son, friend, and worker.

Questions

1. Describe how you would grade transferring tasks to facilitate George's abilities/participation.

2. What are some purposeful activities that George could engage in while in long sitting in preparation for lower body dressing?

3. Design your treatment session to assess medication management with George.

4. How would you facilitate George's planning of a successful day trip with his son Matthew?

5. George enters the therapy clinic, and as you are helping him to transfer onto the mat you notice that his pressure relief cushion in his power wheelchair appears flat. What are your next steps and responsibilities?

6. After you help George perform skin inspection, you and he observe that his healed pressure ulcers have been compromised and have re-opened. Again, what is your responsibility as a practitioner in this situation?

7. You know that George has residual higher-level cognitive deficits. Regarding return to driving, what are some areas of concern that you will need to address, including adaptive controls and switches?

8. During your training session between George and his PCA, you become uncomfortable with the way that George and his PCA interact because it seems both verbally and physically abusive. How would you facilitate improvement in their caregiving relationship?

9. After trying to facilitate a healthier relationship between George and his PCA, you determine that George's safety may be in jeopardy. What would you say or do next?

Larry

Outpatient Rehabilitation: Drivers Rehabilitation

Level of Difficulty: Difficult

Overview: Requires an understanding of driving and community mobility for a person after stroke rehabilitation, specifically an understanding of component skills necessary for return to safe driving and how to handle a situation when return to driving is not indicated

Engagement in Occupation to Support Participation in Context(s)

Performance in Areas of Occupation: Spouse and retiree

Primary Impairments and Functional Deficits: Depth perception, visual processing speed, reaction time, attention (e.g., divided, selective, and sustained), ability to follow instructions safely, ability to change lanes safely, ability to navigate intersections safely, insight into deficits

Context: Retiree adamant in resuming independence through driving

Occupational Profile

Larry is a 67-year-old man who sustained a stroke a few months ago. He had an uncomplicated medical course. He participated in acute rehabilitation, home health, and outpatient rehabilitation to address limitations in his ability to participate fully in his community.

Although Larry notices that it takes him longer to do things, he does not see that he is much different from before he had his stroke. He is eager to return to driving so that he does not have to rely on his spouse so much to get out of their house. Larry presents for further outpatient therapy evaluation and treatment specific to the instrumental activities of daily living skills necessary for safe driving. Larry is to be evaluated by the outpatient practitioner regarding pre-driving skills, and then he will participate in a behind-the-wheel evaluation.

Observed Performance in Desired Occupation/Activity

Instrumental Activities of Daily Living

Community Mobility: Currently, Larry has been told to refrain from driving pending further evaluation. His spouse has assumed primary responsibility for driving wherever they need to go in the community. Larry is also able to use public transportation such as the bus system, but he chooses not to use the bus all that frequently and instead stays at home a lot and feels isolated.

The outpatient OT performs a series of evaluations to look at Larry's cognitive, physical, and emotional function related to driving. Here are the findings from the pre-driving screen. Note that results from the screen are only to provide an indication regarding safety with driving, while the most accurate results regarding ability to return to driving would be from a behind-the-wheel evaluation on the road by a practitioner with driving specialty certification.

Clinical Results in Preparation for Behind the Wheel Testing

Currently driving?   *Not in the last 2 months.*

Restrictions?   *None.*

Any accidents in the last 3 years?   *2 in the last 6 months.*
Evidence of seizures?   *No.*
Medications?   *Blood pressure and cholesterol.*

Pre-Vehicle Assessment				
Physical Skills	**Right Upper Extremity**	**Left Upper Extremity**	**Right Lower Extremity**	**Left Lower Extremity**
Strength	within functional limits	within functional limits	within functional limits	within functional limits
Coordination	within functional limits	within functional limits	within functional limits	within functional limits
Range of Motion	within functional limits	within functional limits	within functional limits	within functional limits
Sensation/ Proprioception	within functional limits	within functional limits	within functional limits	within functional limits
	Within Functional Limits		**Below Functional Limits**	
Neck Rotation	✔			
Sitting Balance	✔			
Standing Balance	✔			
Endurance	✔			

(Continues)

Pre-Vehicle Assessment *(Continued)*		
Wheelchair Mobility (manual or power)	Not Applicable	
Ambulation	Larry is able to ambulate moderate to long distances using a straight end cane.	
Transfers	Larry is able to perform transfers with independence.	
Visual Skills	**Yes**	**No**
Glasses/ Contacts	✔	
	Within Functional Limits	**Below Functional Limits**
Visual Field (peripheral)	130 ✔	
Acuity	left eye 20/30 right eye 20/80 both eyes 20/30 ✔	
Color Discrimination	✔	
Traffic Sign Recognition (x/12 Correct)	12/12 ✔	
Stereopsis/ Depth Perception		✔
Contrast Sensitivity	✔	
Cognitive/ Perceptual Skills	**Within Functional Limits**	**Below Functional Limits**
Visual Processing Speed		✔
Visual Memory	✔	
Short Blessed Test (dementia screen) Score of 8 or above indicates dementia	7 ✔	
Symbol Digit Score of 25 or less indicates concerns with driving		12 ✔

(Continues)

Pre-Vehicle Assessment	(Continued)		
Weintraub Structured Array	**Random, but 0 errors** ✔		
Dynavision			
	Mode A	15	Score of 52+ considered safe driver
	Mode B	3	Score of 42+ considered safe driver
	Divided Attention	16	Score of 35+ considered safe driver
	Continuous (4 minute)	93	Score of 200+ considered safe driver
	Within Functional Limits		**Below Functional Limits**
Ability to Follow Instructions			✔
Insight			✔
Useful Field of View			
	Crash Risk		**5 High Risk**
	Central Vision/ Processing Speed		**Difficulty**
	Divided Attention		**Severe Difficulty**
	Selective Attention		**Difficulty**
Hearing	**Intact**		
Hearing Aids	**No**		
Driving Simulator	Larry was able to put on his seat belt, adjust the seat, and start the car well. He was able to apply both the accelerator and brake effectively. He was able to turn the steering wheel accurately. He was inconsistently able to follow directions from the trainer on the simulator especially in staying in the left lane. He frequently ended up speeding. Larry had difficulties at intersections, especially when turning left or waiting for pedestrians.		

In-Vehicle Assessment Pre-Road Performance		
	Within Functional Limits	Below Functional Limits
Unlock/Lock Doors	✔	
Entry/Exit of Vehicle	✔	
Adjustment of Seat	✔	
Adjustment of Mirrors	✔	
Seat Belt Use	✔	
Operation of Accelerator/Brake	✔	
Reaction Time of Gas to Brake	✔	
Operation of Steering	✔	
Operation of Secondary Controls	✔	

Type of vehicle used ⟨**Sedan**⟩ Mini-Van Full Size Van Other
Seating ⟨**Regular**⟩ Wheelchair Torso Support Extra Cushions Other
Adaptive Equipment Used:⟨**None**⟩
Mechanical Hand Control (type:)
Steering Device (type:)
Left Foot Accelerator
Gas/Brake Block
Right-Hand Turn Signal
Modified Secondary Controls (specify:)
Other: (specify:)

On-the-Road Performance			
Vehicle Operation		**Within Functional Limits**	**Below Functional Limits**
	Acceleration/ Braking	✔	
	Steering/Vehicle Tracking	✔	
	Right Turns	✔	
	Left Turns	✔	
	Parking and Backing Maneuvers	✔	
Traffic Flow		**Within Functional Limits**	**Below Functional Limits**
	Speed Adjustment	✔	
	Lane Changing/ Merging		✔
	Vehicle Spacing, Following Distance	✔	
	Positioning/Speed for Stopping	✔	
	Techniques/ Procedures at Intersections		✔
Scanning and Observation Techniques		**Within Functional Limits**	**Below Functional Limits**
	Use of Mirrors		✔
	Checking Blind Spots		✔
	Identification/ Compliance with Signs	✔	
	Dynamic Scanning of Environment		✔
	Uncontrolled Intersections		✔

(Continues)

On-the-Road Performance *(Continued)*			
Concentration/ Attention to Driving Task		**Within Functional Limits**	**Below Functional Limits**
	Managing Distractions		✔
	Accommodating to Unpredictable Change	✔	
	Anticipation/ Planning in Traffic	✔	
	Sustained Attention	✔	
	Attending to Multiple Stimuli		✔
		Within Functional Limits	**Below Functional Limits**
Perceived Risk			✔
Path Finding Skills		✔	
Knowledge of Traffic Rules		✔	
Judgment/ Decision Making			✔
Emotional Response			✔
Freeway/ Highway Driving	**Not Tested secondary to poor performance on previous on-the-road testing**	**Within Functional Limits**	**Below Functional Limits**
	Entering/Exiting		
	Lane Changing/ Merging		
	Speed Adjustment		
	Positioning/Spacing		
	Awareness of Traffic		

Recommendations/ Summary

This client does not demonstrate the ability to safely operate a motor vehicle. Therefore, driving is not recommended at this time.

Synthesis of Abilities and Deficits

Facilitators to Occupational Performance

Larry demonstrates good physical ability regarding component skills necessary for return to driving. His vision is intact, and although he demonstrates decreased organization with scanning he is able to identify specific symbols and road signs accurately. During the on-the-road performance, Larry demonstrates adequate skills related to operating the vehicle.

Barriers to Occupational Performance

Larry demonstrates decreased reaction time, sustained attention, divided attention, and selective attention, which are vital component skills necessary for return to driving. His performance on the driving screen indicates high likelihood that he would be an unsafe driver with risk of crashing his vehicle or causing an accident. During the on-the-road testing, Larry demonstrates decreased ability to manage distractions, pay attention to multiple stimuli, and use mirrors and check for blind spots. Larry demonstrates little insight into his deficits, making it a challenge to work on improving these areas or even discussing alternatives to driving for community mobility. All of these areas contribute to barriers to a successful outcome.

Intervention Implementation

Therapeutic Use of Occupations and Activities

Occupation-Based Activities

Community mobility
Driving
Alternative transportation

Purposeful Activities

Reaction time

Divided attention

Sustained attention

Selective attention

Managing a task with distractions

Checking blind spots and using mirrors to find items

Dynamic scanning

Lane changing

Consultation Process

Collaborate to determine alternative transportation for successful community mobility

Education Process

Provide education about results of on-the-road driving evaluation and recommendations on driving

Intervention Review

Daily informal meetings set with OT to review progress, review treatment plan, and make modifications as needed.

Outcomes

Larry is adamant that he return to driving as soon as possible.

Larry has an anticipated duration of treatment 1 week, with an estimated frequency of 1 to 2 sessions. By the time of discharge, Larry will demonstrate the following:

1. Good understanding of recommendations regarding return to driving

2. Identification of one or two alternatives to driving for safe and successful participation in community mobility

3. Good understanding of home exercise program to work on increasing deficit areas related to component skills of driving

Questions

1. Larry is adamant that the criteria used to determine that he was an unsafe driver were unfair. What is your response both to Larry and to Larry's doctor?

2. From the on-the-road assessment, you determine that Larry's primary difficulties are related to poor observational awareness. What could you incorporate into your treatment sessions to attempt to improve his observational skills, especially related to driving?

3. What specific tasks might you incorporate into treatment to work on improving reaction time?

4. Larry becomes combative at the end of your on-the-road session. What do you do?

5. What would your discussion be like regarding education about alternative resources for community mobility in Larry's area?

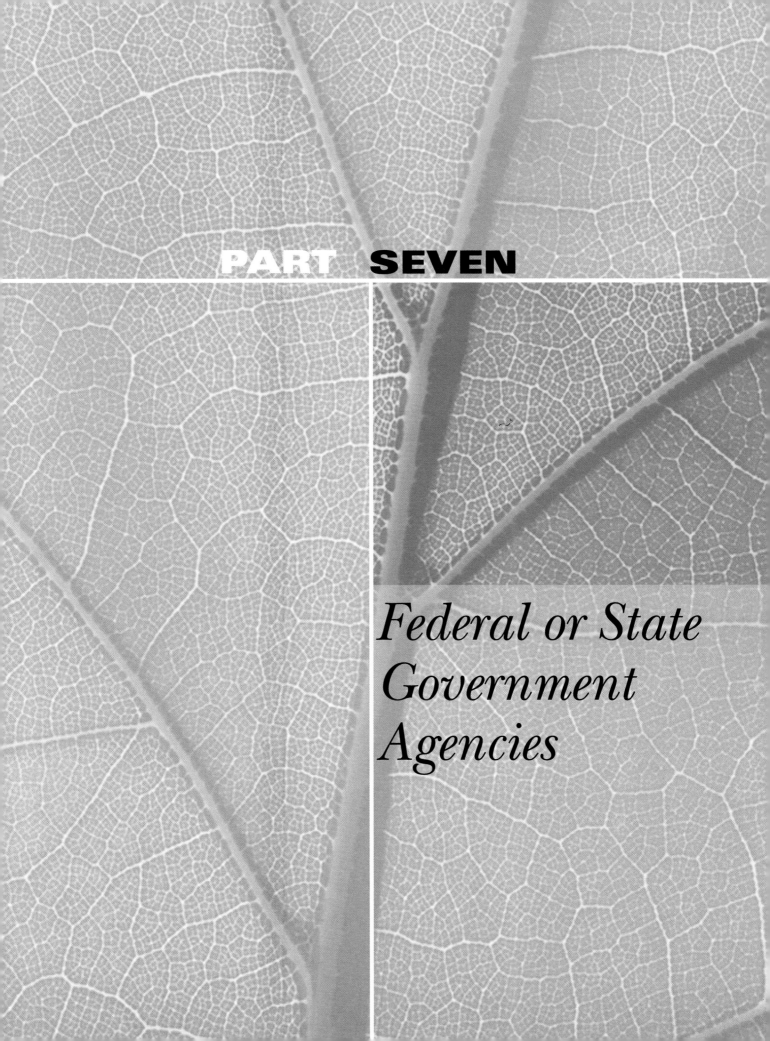

PART SEVEN

Federal or State Government Agencies

Tina

FEDERAL OR STATE GOVERNMENT AGENCIES

Level of Difficulty: Easy

Overview: Requires understanding of the professional code of conduct and scope of practice of an OT assistant, also the understanding of participation in board review of disciplinary action for a COTA

Engagement in Occupation to Support Participation in Context(s)

Context: Certified occupational therapy assistant (COTA) who is under review for complaint of negligence

The following case study does not fit the format of the other cases regarding occupational profile and occupational performance. It involves being a committee member of a state regulatory agency. You are responsible for the review, investigation, and recommendations regarding disciplinary action against a COTA.

General Regulatory Agency Board Questions

1. What types of OTA services are considered unlawful?

2. What credentials are necessary for qualified practice as a COTA?

3. What are the benefits or costs to maintaining registration and credentials through the National Board for Certification in Occupational Therapy?

4. What is the scope of practice of a COTA regarding supervision, ability to complete initial assessments and discharges, and participation in a management role?

5. What are the various types of disciplinary action and options for regaining status to practice as a COTA?

Specific Regulatory Case of COTA Negligence

You and the board are dealing with investigation of a complaint related to negligence. The complaint of negligence is coming from the family of the client because the client continues to be incapable of self-advocating due to cognitive impairments.

Upon investigation, you and the other members of the regulatory board find the following facts:

- The client had sustained a traumatic brain injury resulting in spasticity, decreased sensation, moderate to severe cognitive impairments, decreased mobility, and dependence in self-care.

- The client resided in an inpatient rehabilitation setting for 2 months. Tina, a certified occupational therapy assistant (COTA), provided treatment during this time.
- Tina has over 15 years of experience in treatment of clients with traumatic brain injury.
- Tina had ample access to supervision and collaboration with a group of occupational therapists.
- Over the course of treatment, Tina performed various treatment interventions within her scope of practice.
- The treatment plan included serial casting, splinting, and use of physical agent modalities (e.g., heat, neuromuscular electrical stimulation).
- Looking at Tina's continuing education records, you find that she never completed a physical agent modalities course and is not licensed to practice using physical agent modalities (PAMS) in her state.
- You also find that she did not attend any courses on serial casting.
- Interview of co-workers reveals that Tina received on-the-job training in serial casting with initial close supervision by an OT and was deemed competent.
- The client was found to have pressure sores related to the serial casting that were not reported immediately to the physician and nursing staff.
- As a result of delayed report, the sores became infected, requiring surgical and antibiotic management. This resulted in increased medical costs and length of stay for the client.

Questions

1. What would your recommendations be regarding the allegations of negligence? Please explain your rationale.

2. How would you propose to protect the client while still fostering continued ability to practice as a COTA in the inpatient rehabilitation setting?

3. What additional findings would cause you to recommend a stronger sanction (e.g., suspension or revocation) regarding Tina's code of conduct?

4. Would you modify your recommendations if you found information to support that the COTA reported the pressure sore from the serial cast to the medical staff promptly and documented the information in the medical chart? Why or why not?

References

Minnesota Department of Health. Assuring Competent Care from Qualified Occupational Therapists and Occupational Therapy Assistants: A Consumer Guide to Information and Rights Protected by Law. Retrieved October 17, 2008, from http://www.health.state.mn.us/divs/hpsc/hop/

NBCOT® (February 7, 2003). NBCOT® Candidate/Certificant Code of Conduct. Retrieved October 17, 2008, from http://www.NBCOT.org

NBCOT® (October 2004). Guidelines for Disciplinary Monitoring: NBCOT Remediation Secondary to Disciplinary Action. Retrieved October 17, 2008, from http://www.NBCOT.org

NBCOT® (November 2007). Procedures for the Enforcement of the NBCOT® Candidate/Certificant Code of Conduct. Retrieved October 17, 2008, from http://www.NBCOT.org

Joe

FEDERAL OR STATE GOVERNMENT AGENCIES

Level of Difficulty: Difficult

Overview: Requires understanding of treatment of a soldier who has sustained poly-trauma including traumatic brain injury and is receiving care in a Warrior Transition Unit with the goal of return to military duty or training for productive entry into the community as a veteran

Engagement in Occupation to Support Participation in Context(s)

Performance in Areas of Occupation: Private in the army, spouse, father, and adult son

Primary Impairments and Functional Deficits: Decreased higher-level cognitive function, decreased military combat skills, compromised skin integrity, decreased range of motion, decreased mobility, decreased understanding regarding amputation, burns, and brain injury

Context: 23-year-old married private in the army injured while on a mission who is a new father

Occupational Profile

Joe is a 23-year-old private in the army who was on a mission as a part of Operation Iraqi Freedom in Baghdad, Iraq, when he sustained poly-trauma as the result of the explosion of an improvised explosive device (IED).

Joe and his unit were going from house to house on foot to check for members of Al-Qaeda to increase security for the Iraqi people so that they could go to work and school without worry about being attacked. Joe stepped on a booby-trapped IED which then exploded, injuring Joe and another member of the unit and killing two others. Joe had received training in first aid, was aware of the possibility of IEDs in the area, and most importantly was wearing his flak jacket, so his injuries were less severe than they could have been. His main injuries were caused by the pressure wave of the primary blast, by penetrating and non-penetrating wounds of the secondary blast, and from being thrown a distance. There was a medic on location that was well trained in what injuries to look for after an IED explosion. Joe was quickly stabilized in emergency and then sent to Walter Reed Medical Hospital for surgery and medical management.

Joe is married and recently became a father for the first time; his daughter was born while he was in Iraq. His spouse remains on maternity leave at this time although she has periodic help from her parents. Joe was the primary breadwinner and is concerned about his ability to return to active duty to provide for his growing family.

After surgery and medical stabilization, Joe remains with a mild brain injury, burns to his right hand and arm, and a transtibial amputation to his right leg. The medical doctor suspects that Joe's recovery and healing is going to require greater than 6 months of treatment. For this reason, Joe is being admitted to a Warrior Transition Unit (WTU) where his primary mission can be to heal.

A Warrior Support Triad of a squad leader, nurse case manager, and primary care manager (physician) coordinate Joe's care at the WTU. The WTU further includes an integrated team of professionals: OT, PT, social workers, speech language pathologists, and chaplain. As needed, additional specialists from the Military Treatment Facility will be available to support the medical, behavioral, health, and physical needs of Joe.

Joe will participate in various phases of care while at the WTU. The phases of care in the WTU include these six: *inprocessing* (entrance into WTU with transition to previous roles while receiving medical and rehabilitation care along with housing, administrative, and financial assistance), *assessment* (evaluation of level of function including military job skills and training, interests, and abilities), *goal setting* (establishment of goals related to healing of heart, mind, body, and spirit), *rehabilitation* (focus on treatment to increase ability level and individualized needs), *transition preparation* (discharge planning to leave as either soldier or veteran), and *transition/post-transition* (follow up appointments to facilitate smooth reentry to the military or community).

While in the WTU, Joe will be assigned quarters and treatment with progression through four tiers of rehabilitation: *Tier A* (medical recovery and rest), *Tier B* (basic rehabilitation and reset for return to mission capability with education and training), *Tier C* (participate in targeted interventions including behavioral health strategies, life skills, pain management, cognitive retraining, biofeedback, adaptive skills, vocational rehabilitation, and assistance with work placement), and *Tier D* (resume more normal schedule involved in therapeutic work activities, educational activities, or vocational training activities).

Analysis of Occupational Performance

Synthesis of Occupational Profile

Joe is a 23-year-old married private who is a new father who sustained a mild traumatic brain injury, burns, and right transtibial amputation during an operation in Iraq when an improvised explosive device blew up. He was flown to Walter Reed Medical Center for surgery and medical management of his poly-trauma. He was stabilized and is now assigned quarters and treatment at the local Warrior Transition Unit with focus on fostering healing and either return to active duty or transition to alternative productive activity as a civilian.

Observed Performance in Desired Occupation/Activity

Activities of Daily Living

Bathing: Joe requires maximal assistance for bathing in a roll-in shower. Joe has had a difficult time looking at his body since the explosion. He has to have his right hand covered to protect the healing skin grafts. His residual limb also needs to be covered so that the incision is not compromised. He is unable to stand for the shower and needs to sit on a rolling shower chair.

Bowel and Bladder Management: Because of decreased mobility, Joe is having problems with constipation and needs to have a suppository every few days. He is not having bladder problems. However, because of difficulty with transfers, he has had trouble getting to the toilet in time and has had a few bladder accidents, which he finds extremely embarrassing.

Dressing: Joe requires moderate assistance for putting on a T-shirt. He is currently unable to put on such clothing as his uniform because he cannot manage buttons. Joe is dependent for lower body dressing because he cannot help enough to be performing 25% or more of the task. He is unable to stand on his left leg without increased assistance at this time so he has been getting help to get dressed from a bed level. Joe wants to be able to wear his boots, but he cannot manage them at this time.

Eating/Feeding: Joe is feeding himself with his non-dominant hand. He needs help to open containers and cut food. He does not have any modifications to his diet.

Grooming: Joe requires moderate assistance for grooming from a seated position. Because he is not able to use his dominant hand at this time, Joe is requesting assistance to shave. He needs help to clean his right hand because of the burns.

Functional Mobility: Joe requires maximal assistance for his overall functional mobility. Joe needs moderate assistance to roll from side to side and maximal assistance to go from supine to sit. He is able to go from sitting to supine with minimal assistance. Joe is able to help with a sit pivot transfer from bed to a wheelchair, but he needs repetition and cues for technique and safety. He is able to stand on his left leg at the parallel bars with maximal assistance. He is using a manual wheelchair, but he cannot propel it independently at this time.

Sexual Activity: Joe is concerned that he will have difficulty in sexual performance with his spouse. He is further concerned about how she will see him with his burns and amputation.

Sleep/Rest: Joe tends to sleep a lot during the day and is awake and restless in the middle of night.

Toilet Hygiene: Joe is dependent for tasks related to clothing management and hygiene. He is unable to stand without maximal assistance and then cannot let go of a rail to manage his clothing for toileting. He is not able to wipe thoroughly after a bowel movement using his non-dominant hand, and he is not supposed to use his right hand while the skin grafts are healing.

Instrumental Activities of Daily Living

Community Mobility: Before the explosion, Joe drove. He is currently unable to walk or drive in the WTU without assistance.

Health Management and Maintenance: As a part of being a private in the army, Joe received regular medical care. Until now, he has been extremely healthy and has never had to stay in a hospital overnight. Joe's brain injury has caused him to have difficulty remembering what medications he is taking, when to take them, and what they are for. Joe needs close care of his residual limb and burns to his right hand at this time.

Home Establishment and Management: When not in active duty, Joe is responsible for the outside work at his house. He helps to pick up after himself, but his spouse is responsible for the majority of the housework.

Meal Preparation and Cleanup: At home, Joe helps to clean up after meals. His spouse does the cooking.

Education

Formal Educational Participation: Joe joined the army straight out of high school. Joe was an average student in high school.

Work

Job Performance: Joe has been in the army as a private for the past 5 years. He has served two active rotations in Operation Iraqi Freedom. Joe is strong in his desire to be able to return to active duty soon. He demonstrates decreased performance in the following skills for being a soldier: life skills, peak performance, and abilities to complete operations-related duties.

Employment Interests and Pursuits: As stated previously, Joe is resistant to discussing alternative employment interests or pursuits. Other than working at a grocery store during high school, Joe has not held any job other than that of the military. Joe does enjoy working with computers and fixing things.

Leisure

Leisure Exploration and Participation: Joe has not had much time to explore leisure interests or pursuits. He is fully committed to his duty as a private in the army.

Social Participation

Family: Joe is married and his spouse just gave birth to their first daughter while he was in Iraq. Joe's parents live nearby, as do his parents-in-law. Both sets of family have been supportive of Joe's spouse as she cares for their daughter alone.

Peer, Friend: Joe's primary friends are in his military unit, which he would like to get back to soon. The same explosion that wounded Joe killed two of his closest friends and wounded another unit member.

Factors Influencing Performance Skills and Patterns

Motor Skills

Posture: Joe has difficulty with static balance when standing on his left leg, needing to have someone support him while he holds onto a rail tightly. Other than this, he is not having difficulty with his posture or balance.

Mobility: As was stated before, Joe is having difficulty with his mobility. He needs maximal assistance to get into a wheelchair from his bed. He needs moderate assistance to roll from side to side. He is unable to propel a manual wheelchair without assistance because of the bandaging and restricted movements of his right hand. Joe is able to stand with maximal assistance to get up and then can support himself in the parallel bars with minimal assistance for less than a minute.

Coordination: Joe is having difficulty with coordination because of not being able to use his dominant hand at this time.

Strength and Effort: Joe's strength is relatively good at 4+ to 5/5 throughout his upper extremities, but he reports that he feels that he has gotten weak while he has been off duty. He is unable to use his right arm effectively without compromising the healing burns and skin grafts.

Energy: Joe fatigues easily and tends to sleep during the day. He needs rest breaks every 10 minutes when he is awake and attempting to participate in various activities.

Process Skills

Joe has many deficits with his processing skills including the areas of executive function. He has difficulty planning projects and managing time to complete tasks, decreased organization and sequencing, difficulties memorizing and retrieving information, difficulties initiating tasks, and difficulty generating ideas and alternative solutions to problems. Furthermore, Joe has difficulty with attention to detail, divided attention, accurate ability to evaluate ideas and performance, and he does not engage in group-dynamics appropriately.

Communication/Interaction Skills

Joe is having difficulty tracking conversations and knowing how to take turns with others and needs reminders not to interrupt. He can communicate his basic needs, but he loses the ability to articulate himself when the conversation is more abstract.

Habits and Routines

Joe's habits and routines have been disrupted completely. He would like to get back to the routine that he was used to during his convoy missions and basic training. Because Joe has barely seen his new daughter, he is uncertain of the routines and habits necessary for being a successful father.

Factors Influencing Context(s)

Cultural

Joe remains committed to the army and its culture. He values a commitment to duty, honor, and his country, even sometimes at the sacrifice of his family. He believes strongly in following orders of his commanding officers.

Physical

Because of his amputation and burns to his hand, Joe is limited in his mobility and must deal with increasing the accessibility around his home and the military if he hopes to return to active duty. He is hoping to heal quickly and be measured for a prosthesis so that he can ambulate and complete necessary skills to fulfill his duty as a soldier.

Social

Joe's family is supportive especially his spouse. He values the support of his unit and is mourning the loss of two of his closest unit members.

Personal

Joe is a 23-year-old married man who is newly a father and is strongly entrenched in military life.

Synthesis of Abilities and Deficits

Facilitators to Occupational Performance

Joe is motivated to return to active duty even though he will need to have some accommodations because of his amputation. He remains committed to his duty as an officer, while wanting to heal to be able to spend time with his new daughter. Joe's spouse and family are incredibly supportive of him and want to help him to heal and return home. Joe is a part of the WTU, which is a part of the military with the sole mission of helping wounded soldiers heal and either resume active duty or transition into productive civilian life. Joe's brain injury is mild, affecting higher-level executive function problems. Joe's burns are contained to his right arm and hand. Joe has been healthy until this explosion and shows promise of resiliency.

Barriers to Occupational Performance

Joe continues to heal from poly-trauma. He is having difficulties dealing with not being with his military unit, especially after the death of two of his closest unit members. He is having difficulties processing information, memorizing it, and retrieving it. He has limited strength and mobility at this time because of his burns and amputation. Joe is having difficulty seeing any life alternatives other than returning to active military duty.

Intervention

Intervention Plan

Collaborative Client Goals that are Objective and Measurable

Joe would like to return to active duty with his military unit. He would also like to be able to spend time with his spouse and new daughter. He would like to be able to ambulate with a prosthetic limb.

The following goals are established to be specific to helping the healing of Joe's heart, mind, body, and spirit. Joe has an anticipated duration of treatment of greater than 6 months with an estimated frequency of daily OT sessions. By the time of discharge, Joe will perform the following:

1. Demonstrate good understanding of recommendations regarding possibility of returning to military service
2. Demonstrate good understanding of recommendations regarding transitioning to productive civilian life
3. Identify one or two vocational interests plus the resources available to pursue them
4. Follow daily schedule with modified independence using a day planner
5. Demonstrate good understanding of exercise, range of motion, and massage for burn care management
6. Participate in child-rearing activities with his daughter and minimal supervision

By the time of discharge, Joe's family will demonstrate the following:

1. Good understanding of Joe's need for assistance/supervision

Discharge Needs and Plan

Joe wants to be able to return to Iraq once he is cleared medically. However, with the extent of his injuries, this is probably not realistic; therefore discharge is planned for home with family, with focus on identifying alternative employment for achieving productive integration into civilian community. Most likely Joe will still need ongoing outpatient OT services at the time of discharge.

Intervention Implementation

Therapeutic Use of Occupations and Activities

Occupation-Based Activities

Life skills training
    Child rearing
Work reintegration
    Vocational and work programs
    Identification and access of resources

Soldier skill reintegration
    Functional warrior skills evaluation to determine fitness for duty
    Improving and maintaining ability to fire weapon or complete convoy mission
    Battle simulation center
    Engagement skills training center

Time management
    Working within a schedule
    Organizing day

Medication management and health maintenance

Anger management

Leisure exploration and participation

Stress management

Community reintegration

Community mobility
  Driving
  Public transportation
Community outings

Purposeful Activities

Practice loading and unloading firearm in timed setting

Practice donning and doffing uniform, including boots

Create a morning checklist for the day's activities

Write out description of past convoy mission

Practice carrying on a conversation about an assigned topic, including taking turns

Practice changing a diaper

Preparatory Methods

Pain management

Exercise and activity tolerance

Wound and burn care
  Anti-contracture positioning
    Fabricate and use specialized inserts
    Range of motion (daily stretching routines and positioning programs)
  Skin inspection and care
  Desensitization
  Scar management
    Massage
    Pressure therapy

Psychosocial aspects of traumatic event

Consultation Process

Collaborate in the following:

    To determine level of fitness required for return to military duty

    To identify alternative education and work opportunities

Education Process

Educate about the following:

    Basic training topics including sleep hygiene, maintaining a healthy weight after injury, financial benefits and money management, educational benefits and career planning, avoiding addictions, and relationship coaching

    Range of motion, exercise program, splinting, and burn care program

    Wear, care, and purpose of burn garment

    Wound healing and tissue response to exercise and scar management techniques

    Brain injury and compensatory strategies

Intervention Review

Daily informal meetings set with OT to review progress, review treatment plan, and make modifications as needed.

Outcomes

Along with reviewing progress toward Joe's objective goals, therapy will continue to focus on his ability to resume participation in his roles of spouse, father, and private in the army.

Questions

1. You and the OT have determined that Joe does not have the skills to resume active duty. How do you handle the conversation with Joe? Who else from the team might you involve in this discussion and why?

2. Even though you have determined that Joe will be unable to return to active duty, how might you help him to explore options for work that allow him to remain in the military?

3. Pick an activity from the list of ideas above and show how you would grade the task for both level of skill and reduction in cognitive cues.

4. While teaching Joe skin inspection, you notice that his residual limb is a different color, has increased drainage, and a foul smell. What do you do?

5. How would your treatment plan and approach change based on whether Joe was in the four tiers of rehabilitation in the WTU (Tier A, Tier B, Tier C, and Tier D)?

6. Joe says that his spouse and daughter are coming to visit for the first time and he is both excited and nervous. How would you incorporate the meeting into a successful treatment session to facilitate a positive experience for Joe and his family?

References

Erickson, Mary W., Secrest, Debra S., and Gray, Amy L. (2008). Army Occupational Therapy in the Warrior Transition Unit, July 28.

Globalsecurity.org. (2008). Improvised Explosive Devices (IEDs)/Booby Traps. Retrieved October 28, 2008, from http://www.globalsecurity.org/military/intro/ied.htm

Steele, W.M., and Walters, R.P., Jr. (September/October 2001). Training and Developing Leaders in a Transforming Army. *Military Review*, 2-10.

Tolzman, Michael. (January 24, 2008). Warrior Transition Units' Mission Second Only to Combat, Say Officials. Comprint Military Publications. Retrieved October 17, 2008, from http://www.dcmilitary.com/stories/012408/stripe_28046.shtml

PART EIGHT

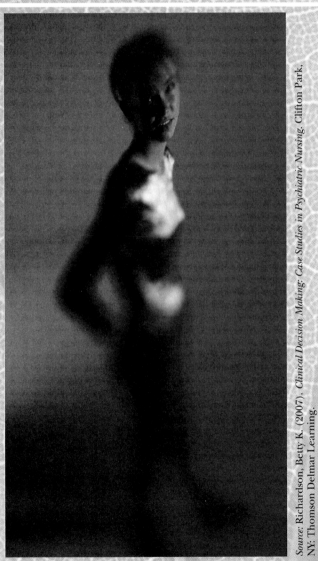

Eating disorders can result in a distorted body image.

Source: Richardson, Betty K. (2007). *Clinical Decision Making: Case Studies in Psychiatric Nursing.* Clifton Park, NY: Thomson Delmar Learning.

Psychiatric Care

Michiko

PSYCHIATRIC CARE

Level of Difficulty: Moderate

Overview: Requires understanding of age-specific considerations along with clinical reasoning skills in the treatment of a teenager with bulimia nervosa in an outpatient psychiatric day program setting

Engagement in Occupation to Support Participation in Context(s)

Performance in Areas of Occupation: Student, dancer, daughter, sister, and friend

Primary Impairments and Functional Deficits: Poor concentration, dizziness, decreased life balance, poor life management skills, poor body image, compulsive exercising and other compensatory behaviors, decreased understanding of nutrition, stressors, and emotional reaction to food and eating

Context: 16-year-old Japanese girl in her junior year of high school heavily involved in school dance troupe

MODERATE

Occupational Profile

Michiko is a 16-year-old girl who is a junior in high school. She presented to the emergency room with complaints of abdominal fullness and dyspnea. She reported that she had overeaten and attempted to vomit but was unsuccessful. Her height and weight were 5 foot 3 inches and 153 pounds. She reported an irregular menstrual cycle. Her abdomen was found to be distended and tender. She had relatively stable vital signs, although further testing revealed that her electrolytes were out of balance. Radiographic views were obtained of her abdomen and she was found to have a large mass consistent with a dilated stomach. A computed tomography (CT) was performed and revealed a cystic mass including homogenous water density contents with floating air bubbles. Large amounts of fluid were aspirated from the stomach using a nasogastric tube. She was thought to be stable, but just before transferring to an acute inpatient psychiatric unit she went into a pre-shock state with increased abdominal pain, cyanosis, and decreased urine output.

Michiko's blood pressure had dropped to 80/60 mmHg and her pulse rate was high. Her abdomen was again severely distended and rigid with increased tenderness. Her bowel sounds were barely audible. Labs were drawn and she was found

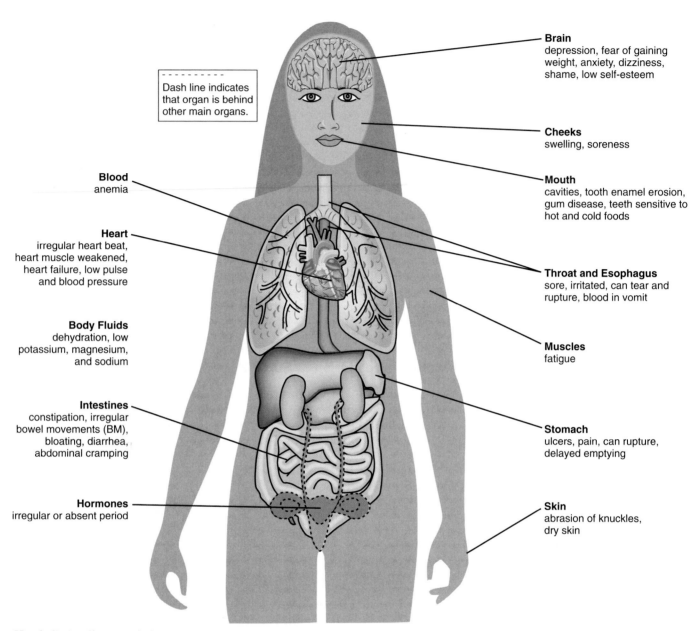

Brain
depression, fear of gaining weight, anxiety, dizziness, shame, low self-esteem

Cheeks
swelling, soreness

Mouth
cavities, tooth enamel erosion, gum disease, teeth sensitive to hot and cold foods

Throat and Esophagus
sore, irritated, can tear and rupture, blood in vomit

Muscles
fatigue

Stomach
ulcers, pain, can rupture, delayed emptying

Skin
abrasion of knuckles, dry skin

Blood
anemia

Heart
irregular heart beat, heart muscle weakened, heart failure, low pulse and blood pressure

Body Fluids
dehydration, low potassium, magnesium, and sodium

Intestines
constipation, irregular bowel movements (BM), bloating, diarrhea, abdominal cramping

Hormones
irregular or absent period

- - - - - - - - - -
Dash line indicates that organ is behind other main organs.

How bulimia affects your body.

to have an elevated white blood cell count. A repeat radiograph demonstrated subphrenic air and she was diagnosed with diffuse peritonitis. She underwent an emergent laparotomy, which revealed a stomach that was dilated with necrotic changes including perforation. The stomach was resected and she was stabilized.

Michiko recovered enough from her surgery without further complications so that she transitioned to acute inpatient psychiatric treatment for 2 weeks. She was discharged to home with her parents with a plan to seek further treatment of her bulimia nervosa.

Michiko has a history of excessive exercising and is an active member of her school dance troupe. She is a junior in high school and used to be a top student. Over the past several months, she has demonstrated a decline in her grades and several unexcused absences. Of note is that Michiko's parents have been going through an intense separation.

Michiko reports an obsession with food and dieting. She states that she is not happy with how she looks compared to the other girls at her school. She reports that she has been increasingly teased about her weight over the past few years of school.

Michiko is now medically stable and has recovered from her surgery. She has been evaluated by acute inpatient psychiatric OT and social work and found to be an excellent candidate for the psychiatric day treatment program. The comprehensive day program is 3 days per week including involvement of an OT, social worker, dietitian and nutrition therapist, psychiatrist, psychologist, and primary care physician.

Analysis of Occupational Performance

Synthesis of Occupational Profile

Michiko is a 16-year-old girl who is a junior in high school. She presented to the emergency hospital with severe complications with electrolyte imbalances and a near heart attack. She was diagnosed with bulimia nervosa. She was medically stabilized and transferred to an inpatient psychiatric unit specializing in eating disorders. She is now back home but needing to attend ongoing therapy to address comprehensive treatment at an outpatient psychiatric day program. She will be attending the program 3 times per week while slowly reintegrating back into her junior year classes. Focus of treatment is to address improved life skills in emotional, physical, and psychological function to enable successful reengagement in roles of student, dancer, daughter, sister, and friend.

Observed Performance in Desired Occupation/Activity

Activities of Daily Living

Bathing: Michiko can be compulsive about cleanliness, taking multiple showers in a given day. She attempts to scrub herself not only to get clean but also to remove her excess weight.

Bowel and Bladder Management: Michiko makes frequent trips to the bathroom. She admits to prolonged use of laxatives to help maintain her weight.

Dressing: Michiko wears loose fitting clothing to hide that she is slightly overweight. She has a distorted self-image of her body type and shape.

Eating/Feeding: Michiko talks constantly about dieting and food. She avoids most foods, stating that they are fattening. When surrounded by others, she tends to eat very small portions. Michiko tends to eat a lot at a given time and then excuses herself to use the bathroom. Schoolteachers have frequently found Michiko vomiting.

Grooming: Michiko takes time to make sure that she looks her best although she reports that she is never satisfied with her appearance. She is able to complete grooming independently, but it takes too much time and sometimes makes her late for things like catching the school bus.

Functional Mobility: Michiko does not have issues with functional mobility, although she does report feeling weak and dizzy at times.

Toileting: Michiko spends her time going to and from the bathroom throughout the school day. She uses laxatives to make sure that she can get rid of food, especially when she feels that she has overeaten. She also has a history of increased vomiting with noticeable scarring along her esophagus from repeated purging.

Instrumental Activities of Daily Living

Care of Pets: Michiko is responsible for feeding the cat and dog. She loves to take her dog on long walks as a part of her daily exercise routine.

Community Mobility: Michiko just completed her driving test and is now able to drive without another person in the car. Unfortunately, she rarely gets access to the family car, so she still uses public transportation to get around.

Health Management and Maintenance: Michiko still sees a pediatrician on an annual basis. She reports that although she grew up with this doctor, he seems out of touch with her needs or those of other teenage girls.

Home Establishment and Management: Michiko has several chores around the house. She tries to keep her room cleaned compulsively, and she has difficulty with any messes. As Michiko's function has declined, she has had less energy or motivation to complete chores other than cleaning.

Meal Preparation and Cleanup: Michiko is obsessed with food and dieting. She likes to make sure that she packs her own meals for school. She avoids many nutritious foods because she feels that they are too fattening. Other than school lunches and breakfast, Michiko's mother makes her meals.

Education

Formal Educational Participation: Michiko is a junior in high school. She used to be a top student, but recently she has been cutting classes and demonstrating a poor attitude about school and schoolwork, and her grades have declined.

Work

Employment Interests and Pursuits: Michiko used to have a part-time job after school, but her parents made her quit after receiving her most recent report card.

Leisure

Leisure Exploration: Michiko does not have time for additional leisure pursuits. However, she does report a need to do things compulsively and an inability to relax and feel happy frequently.

Leisure Participation: Michiko is actively involved in the dance troupe at school. When not dancing, Michiko is committed to exercising for multiple hours at a time. She has difficulty if she is unable to exercise for any reason.

Social Participation

Community: Michiko used to be active in her community through her church, but she has isolated herself from these groups as her function has declined.

Family: Michiko's parents are separated. She has two other siblings and is the middle child of the family. The family also has a cat and a dog. Michiko's parents have been focused on their own dynamics and potential pursuit of divorce. Until recently, they did not observe any dramatic changes in Michiko's behaviors, although they are now quite concerned about her health and safety.

Peer, Friend: Michiko has a few close friends, but she has been isolating herself over the past few months.

Factors Influencing Performance Skills and Patterns

Motor Skills

Posture: Michiko does not have any issues with her postural control.

Mobility: Michiko prides herself on being extremely active. When not participating in dance at school, she exercises daily for hours on end.

Strength and Effort: Michiko is obsessed with achieving a certain weight to enhance her ability to perform in dance at school.

Energy: Michiko reports increased fatigue and dizziness although she still exercises for long periods every day, including participating in dance at school.

Process Skills

Michiko reports decreased ability to concentrate over the past few months. She is having difficulty reacting quickly to information.

Communication/Interaction Skills

Michiko has started isolating herself and reports feeling self-conscious when interacting with her classmates and friends.

Habits and Routines

Michiko has been able to maintain most of her routines, but her obsession with exercise and food has made it more challenging for her to participate fully in her student and friend role.

Roles

Michiko is a student, daughter, sister, friend, and dancer. When she is feeling weaker, she has more difficulty engaging in her role as a dancer. She has been having more academic difficulties with her student role the past few months.

Factors Influencing Context(s)

Cultural

Michiko comes from a middle-class background and is Japanese. There is a cultural value to being thin, and the media frequently reports on the epidemic of obesity around the world.

Physical

There are no physical factors other than personal factors of poor self-image and distortion of body type.

Social

Although Michiko has a few close friends; she has been the target of bullying about her weight and body image by classmates. Over the past several months, Michiko has spent increasing amounts of time alone.

Personal

Michiko is a 16-year-old junior in high school with a strong interest in dancing.

Synthesis of Abilities and Deficits

Facilitators to Occupational Performance

Michiko is aware of the serious nature of being diagnosed with bulimia nervosa. She was very upset and shocked to find that her behaviors had contributed to perforations in her abdomen that required surgery. She hopes that she will be able to regain her ability to participate in school and graduate, and perhaps pursue a dancing career. Although Michiko was critically ill because of her bulimia nervosa, the diagnosis was caught fairly early, with a greater chance of treatment being effective in leading to a healthier outcome.

Barriers to Occupational Performance

The medical nature of Michiko's eating disorder is complicated and critical. Michiko is ambivalent about how successful she will be in conquering her eating disorder. She is aware of the grave nature of her illness, but she has difficulty identifying alternative solutions. She is experiencing negative stress from the separation of her parents and feeling bullied at her school. Although Michiko's parents are concerned about her health and wellness, they have been having their own difficulties because of marital discord.

Intervention

Intervention Plan

Collaborative Client Goals that are Objective and Measurable

Michiko has an anticipated duration of treatment for 3 to 6 months with an estimated frequency of 3 times per week. By the time of discharge, Michiko will perform the following:

1. Demonstrate increased accuracy and positive report of body image through both verbal report and actions

2. Create several healthy meals from start to finish including appropriate portion sizes

3. Engage in one or two relaxation techniques or activities, especially during times of increased stress

4. Demonstrate good understanding of the relationship of stress, vulnerability, and occupational balance

Discharge Needs and Plan

Michiko is planning to return to school next semester at least part-time. Although she is ambivalent about being able to manage her bulimia nervosa in a more healthy way, she hopes to find a healthy balance that allows her to resume activities like participating in the school dance troupe. Michiko, her family, and her teachers and classmates will benefit from education about eating disorders and their effective treatment. By the time of discharge from the day treatment program for people with eating disorders, it is likely that Michiko will continue to benefit from weekly, progressing to monthly, counseling sessions with a psychologist. She will also benefit from having a resource and checklist that can be used after she returns to school in order to help retain functional performance in all of her life roles, especially that of student.

Intervention Implementation

Therapeutic Use of Occupations and Activities

Occupation-Based Activities

Meal planning and preparation

Leisure Exploration and Participation
    Arts and crafts
    Gardening
    Creative writing

School and time management

Purposeful Activities

Participate in components of body image workshop

Identify one or two triggers to binge eating

Identify one or two healthier strategies to deal with reducing stress

Participate in eating one or two lunches per week with other group members

Go on outing to local restaurant

Participate in yoga fitness class

Engage in daily journaling of feelings and actions, especially surrounding meal times

Preparatory Methods

Relaxation techniques

Biofeedback

Cognitive behavioral therapy

Anger management

Stress management

Consultation Process

Collaborate in the following:

Creating a list of symptoms and triggers to binge and purge behaviors

Identifying healthier choices to binge and purge behaviors

Determining more accurate self-awareness of body image

Education Process

Education on the following:

Nutrition and healthier lifestyle

Exercise and striking a healthy balance

Life management skills, including stress reduction and anger management

Family training about bulimia nervosa and treatment strategies effective in restoring healthier engagement in life occupations

Intervention Review

Daily informal meetings set with OT to review progress, review treatment plan, and make modifications as needed.

Outcomes

Along with reviewing progress toward Michiko's objective goals, therapy will focus on her ability to resume participation in her roles as student, dancer, daughter, sister, and friend.

Questions

1. You walk into the room for your first session and find that Michiko is overweight. She does not fit your image of a person with an eating disorder; why is your image incorrect? What could you do to expand your knowledge about signs and symptoms of eating disorders like bulimia nervosa?

2. You arrive at a session and find that a friend is telling Michiko that her eating disorder is not a true illness. What would you say and do?

3. Describe a session where you discuss the reality that Michiko's bulimia is putting her life at risk, including potential for death if she returns to using laxatives and exercising for multiple hours at a time.

4. How might Michiko's eating disorder contribute to decreased cognitive abilities or functioning when she returns to school?

5. Design a treatment session surrounding teaching life skills for Michiko.

6. Create a day treatment schedule, for the week, of topics that you would cover for Michiko and other participants in the day treatment group for people with eating disorders. Give specific examples for each activity.

7. You happen to walk into the bathroom and hear someone attempting to throw up. You realize that the person is Michiko; how do you handle the situation?

References

Creek, Jennifer. (2002). *Occupational Therapy and Mental Health: Principles, Skills, and Practice.* Elsevier Health Sciences. Philadelphia, PA.

ECRI Health Technology Assessment Information Service. (2006). Evidence Report: Bulimia Nervosa: Efficacy of Available Treatments. Retrieved October 19, 2008, from http://www.bulimiaguide.org/static/report_complete.pdf using the search engine Google and key words, "bulimia nervosa treatment and occupational therapy."

Martin, Joan. (2000). *Eating Disorders, Food, and Occupational Therapy.* Whurr Publishers, Ltd. London, England.

NEDA. (2008). The National Eating Disorders Association Educator Toolkit. Retrieved October 17, 2008, from http://www.nationaleatingdisorders.org/uploads/file/toolkits/NEDA-Toolkit-Educators_09-15-08.pdf

Nakao, Atsunori, Isozaki, Hiroshi, Iwagaki, Hiromi, Kanagawa, Taiichiro, Takakura, Norihisa, and Tanaka, Noriaki. (2000). Gastric Perforation Caused by a Bulimic Attack in an Anorexia Nervosa Patient: Report of a Case. *Surgery, Today 30,* 435-437.

South Coast Medical Center. (2005). Behavioral Health Services: Eating Disorders Program. Retrieved October 19, 2008 from http://www.southcoastmedcenter.com/content/services/behavioral/eating_disorders.asp

Lia

PSYCHIATRIC CARE

Level of Difficulty: Difficult

Overview: Requires understanding of cultural and mental health issues and clinical reasoning skills in the treatment of a Hmong adult in an inpatient psychiatric setting

Engagement in Occupation to Support Participation in Context(s)

Performance in Areas of Occupation: Spouse, mother, farmer, and Hmong community member

Primary Impairments and Functional Deficits: Decreased personal grooming and bathing, decreased safe child rearing, decreased performance in work and leisure, decreased communication, auditory hallucinations, thought disorganization, and paranoia

Context: 27-year-old Hmong mother with paranoid schizophrenia committed to an inpatient psychiatric care after killing two of her children to remove evil spirits

Occupational Profile

Lia is a 25-year-old Hmong woman who is in acute psychiatric hospital for management of paranoid schizophrenia.

Lia was found by her spouse in her home, standing with a bloody knife next to the lifeless bodies of two of their children, whom she had stabbed repeatedly. She was singing quietly and muttering to herself. Concerned neighbors contacted the police who then arrested Lia. The court mandated that Lia undergo psychiatric testing which led to a diagnosis of paranoid schizophrenia. It was determined that she was not fit to stand trial and instead was committed to an inpatient psychiatric hospital for treatment of her mental illness.

Lia moved from Laos when she was 15 and does not speak fluent English. She and her spouse remain closely involved in their Hmong culture and community. They live in a house with their extended family and eight children (now six). They work on their family's farm and sell their goods at the local farmers' market.

Lia enjoys taking care of her family, but over the past few years she has become more paranoid, with the persisting symptoms of hallucinations, conceptual disorganization, suspiciousness, and unusual thoughts. She states that she believed that her children were showing signs of evil and she needed to help to rid them of their evil spirits.

A psychiatrist and psychologist are seeing Lia. She has been started on antipsychotic medication. While in the acute psychiatric hospital, she will also be seen by OT, nursing, and CM services.

Analysis of Occupational Performance

Synthesis of Occupational Profile

Lia is a 25-year-old Hmong woman who has been diagnosed with paranoid schizophrenia that resulted in her killing two of her children. She was found to need intense psychiatric treatment, including medications and supportive therapies. She would benefit from OT services to address improved function in living skills such as basic conversation, recreation for leisure, medication management, and symptom management. It is not certain whether she will be safe to return home to resume her roles as spouse, mother, farmer, and Hmong community member.

Observed Performance in Desired Occupation/Activity

Activities of Daily Living

Bathing: Lia's family reports that she had stopped bathing during the past several weeks. She needs reminders to wash herself.

Bowel and Bladder Management: Lia does not have issues with bowel and bladder management other than feeling as if these functions represent evil spirits coming out of her.

Dressing: Lia is able to dress herself, but she tends not to change her clothes unless reminded that it is an expectation. Her clothing contributes to her disheveled appearance.

Eating/Feeding: Lia does not have any issues with eating, although she has been known to forget to eat, especially when auditory hallucinations are intense and frequent.

Grooming: Lia's appearance is disheveled and she has difficulty with keeping herself well-groomed. She needs reminders to attend better to her overall cleanliness and appearance.

Functional Mobility: Lia does not have any issues with functional mobility.

Toileting: Lia does not have problems with toileting, although she does report that it is a way of purging evil from her body.

Instrumental Activities of Daily Living

Child Rearing: As Lia's illness has progressed; she has become less able to take care of her children safely. She is concerned that she will not be able to return home and take care of them again. She is aware that she stabbed two of her children to death, but she still states that they had evil spirits and that was the only way for her to get rid of them.

Community Mobility: Lia does not drive. She either runs errands with her spouse or takes public transportation. As her illness progressed, she had more difficulties riding on the bus and train because she was convinced that people were watching and talking about her.

Health Management and Maintenance: Lia and her family tend to seek out use of the local shaman before going to the hospital although they do have a primary care physician whom they see annually. Until now, she had not received treatment for her mental illness. She is unfamiliar with taking medications.

Home Establishment and Management and Financial Management: Lia is responsible for paying bills and cleaning the house. She has had increased difficulty with these responsibilities over the past several months. Lia's spouse reports that he just found out that many bills have been left unpaid and that they are at risk for having utilities turned off at their home.

Meal Preparation and Cleanup: Lia rotates with the other women of the house in preparing meals and cleaning up. She has had more difficulties with cooking and cleaning up, especially because of her increased disorganization.

Education

Formal Educational Participation: Lia did not have any formal education because she was needed on the family farm. She does report that it might be helpful to learn more English, especially to communicate with customers at the farmers' market.

Work

Employment Interests and Pursuits: Lia and her family run a farm and sell their produce at the farmers' market. She has had difficulty participating in her responsibilities on the farm over the past several months. She was having difficulty staying organized and on task, especially as her auditory hallucinations became stronger.

Leisure

Leisure Exploration and Participation: Lia does not have many leisure interests, as all of her time when she was healthy was spent raising her children, working on the farm, or completing tasks around the house.

Social Participation

Community: Lia and her family are active members of the Hmong community. As her illness has progressed, Lia has withdrawn from participating in the community. The Hmong community does not understand or recognize mental illness. Instead, they believe that the behaviors are because of evil spirits that have entered a person's body. The Hmong community still values and uses the services of a local shaman to provide healing in combination with Western medicine.

Family: Lia lives with her spouse, remaining six children, and two other families on her spouse's side. Family support is strong, although they are having difficulty understanding what paranoid schizophrenia is and how it is affecting Lia.

Peer, Friend: Lia has kept to her family and to herself over the past several months. She does have friends from the Hmong community in her area, but has been withdrawn from their support.

Factors Influencing Performance Skills and Patterns

Motor Skills

Posture: Lia does not have problems with her postural control.

Mobility: Lia's mobility is not affected by her paranoid schizophrenia.

Coordination: Lia does not have issues with her coordination.

Strength and Effort: Lia's strength has not been affected by her mental illness.

Energy: Lia tends to isolate herself and keep occupied with watching television so that she does not have to listen to the voices in her head. She has not had energy to complete many activities at home for the past several months.

Process Skills

Lia has difficulty separating reality from her delusional thoughts. Her thoughts, although fast paced, are disorganized.

Communication/Interaction Skills

Lia avoids interacting with others. When she does communicate, she is unable to carry on a lengthy conversation that makes any sense. She avoids eye contact. She is still frequently convinced that people are out to get her.

Habits and Routines

Lia's thought disorganization and auditory hallucinations have made it challenging to stay engaged in healthier habits and routines.

Roles

Lia is a mother, spouse, farmer, and community member. As her illness has progressed, she has isolated herself from her community and family. She has not been able to carry out her roles effectively, as indicated by her paranoid behaviors resulting in the murder of her 2 children because she believed they had evil spirits and a voice told her to cut out the evil.

Factors Influencing Context(s)

Cultural

Lia did not move to the United States until she was 18. She and her spouse have been involved in their Hmong community and traditions of their people. The

Hmong culture attempts to blend both Hmong medicine and Western medicine. There is not a word for mental illness in their language. When people behave like Lia, it is typical to involve the local shaman to help rid the person of evil spirits.

Physical

There are no foreseeable physical factors influencing Lia's treatment plan and potential for managing her paranoid schizophrenia.

Social

As stated before, Lia was involved as a Hmong community member, but as she became sicker she withdrew from this social support. Her family is supportive of helping her heal, but they are not completely trusting and understanding of Western medicine.

Personal

Lia is a 27-year-old Hmong mother of six children who works on the family farm growing and selling produce for a living.

Synthesis of Abilities and Deficits

Facilitators to Occupational Performance

Lia was just diagnosed with paranoid schizophrenia; the hope is that the illness was caught early and can be managed successfully. She is motivated to return home to take care of her children and work on the farm. Occasionally, she realizes that she is having auditory hallucinations and thought disorganization. Lia's family is supportive of learning how to help her get better and return home as long as she is not a threat to herself or the other children.

Barriers to Occupational Performance

Lia has difficulty determining what is real versus a hallucination. She has had several months of declining function that has been untreated. The severity of her illness contributed to the death of two of her children. It is uncertain that she will ever be considered safe enough to return to take care of the rest of her children. Although Lia and her family are interested in pursuing treatment to help her, they are skeptical of Western medicine and believe that she is still possessed by evil spirits.

Intervention

Intervention Plan

Collaborative Client Goals that are Objective and Measurable

Lia states that she needs to get back home, but she is not thinking logically enough to articulate realistic goals. Lia's spouse would like to have the evil spirit leave his spouse and for her to return home and be safe with their children.

Lia has an anticipated duration of treatment of 2 to 4 weeks with individual and group OT sessions 3 times per week. By the time of discharge, Lia will perform the following:

1. Practice initiating conversation with others during group sessions and mealtimes
2. Plan and prepare a hot meal with good safety awareness and minimal supervision
3. Increase ability to bathe and groom appropriately to one general reminder per day
4. Organize and follow medication routine for day with minimal cues

By the time of discharge, Lia's family will demonstrate the following:

1. Basic understanding of schizophrenia including identification of symptoms and areas of concern
2. Good understanding of Lia's need for assistance/supervision

Discharge Needs and Plan

Lia would like to return home, but it is uncertain whether she will be considered safe for returning to taking care of her remaining six children. Part of her stay in the inpatient psychiatric hospital will involve determination of safety to herself and others and the ability to return home.

Intervention Implementation
Therapeutic Use of Occupations and Activities

Occupation-Based Activities
Bathing

Personal grooming and personal appearance

Child rearing

Food preparation

Health maintenance

Money management

Transportation

Leisure and recreation

Job maintenance

Purposeful Activities
Practice setting up weekly medications in containers

Practice basic conversation skills

Select and complete simple craft project

Practice cutting up vegetables for a meal

Play a game with her children in controlled, supervised setting

Complete bill-paying task

Consultation Process

Collaborate with client and family to determine the following:

    Safest plan for discharge home

    Leisure options to help with management of negative symptoms

Education Process

Provide education and training about the following:

    Paranoid schizophrenia, its symptoms, and treatment options

    Independent living skills

    Activities known to mediate supportive psychological/psychiatric therapy

Intervention Review

Daily informal meetings set with OT to review progress, review treatment plan, and make modifications as needed.

Outcomes

Along with reviewing progress toward Lia's objective goals, therapy will focus on her ability to resume participation in her roles as spouse, mother, farmer, and community member.

Questions

1. Lia's family informs you that they are bringing in a local shaman to help rid her of her evil spirits. What would your response to the family be?

2. You feel that Lia's interpreter is not sharing complete details with you. How do you approach the interpreter or what would you say to the interpreter's agency?

3. You enter the room and realize that Lia is experiencing increased hallucinations and thought disorganization. What would you do to help Lia? What is your responsibility to other members of the team?

4. You feel strongly that Lia does not deserve to explore treatment options because she killed two of her children. How do you overcome these feelings to provide fair and appropriate care to Lia?

5. You have read several articles that state that expressive therapy is less effective than teaching independent living skills. Why do you think that this would be the case with helping someone like Lia to overcome negative symptoms of her paranoid schizophrenia?

6. How would you help to determine whether Lia is safe to return home with her remaining children?

7. Lia has numerous family members visiting, and their presence appears to be detracting from your therapy sessions. How would you handle this situation?

References

Fadiman, Anne. (1997). *The Spirit Catches You and You Fall Down*. Farrar, Strauss, & Giroux. New York, NY.

Goetz, Kaomi. (August 27, 2001). *Hmong Face Cultural Hurdles to Mental Health Care*. Minnesota Public Radio.

Liberman, R.P., Wallace, C.J., Blackwell, G., Kopelowicz, A., Vaccaro, J.V., and Mintz, J. (1998). Skills Training Versus Psychosocial Occupational Therapy for Persons with Persistent Schizophrenia. *American Journal of Psychiatry*, 155(8), 1087-1091.

Picchioni, M.M., and Murray, R. (2008). Schizophrenia. *Scholarpedia*, 3(4), 4132. http://www.scholarpedia.org/article/Schizophrenia#Positive_symptoms

General References

American Geriatric Society. (2001). Special Series: Clinical Practice. Guidelines for the Prevention of Falls in Older Persons. *Journal of the American Geriatric Society, 49,* 664–672.

American Occupational Therapy Association. (1994). Uniform Terminology for Occupational Therapy—Third Edition. *American Journal of Occupational Therapy, 48,* 1047–1054.

American Occupational Therapy Association. (2003). Tips for Living: Fall Prevention for People with Disabilities and Older Adults. AOTA. Bethesda, MD.

American Occupational Therapy Association. (2003). Tips for Living: Modifying Your Home for Independence. AOTA. Bethesda, MD.

American Occupational Therapy Association. (2004). Definition of Occupational Therapy Practice for the AOTA Model Practice Act. AOTA. Bethesda, MD.

American Occupational Therapy Association. (2008). Occupational Therapy Practice Framework: Domain and Process—Second Edition. *American Journal of Occupational Therapy, 62*(6), 625–688.

Berg, K.O. (1989). Balance and Its Measure in the Elderly: A Review. *Physiotherapy Canada, 41,* 240–246.

Bergen, D. (Ed.). (1988). *Play as a Medium for Learning and Development: A Handbook of Theory and Practice.* Heinemann. Portsmouth, NH.

Borg Perceived Exertion Scale. Retrieved April 4, 2009, from http://www.doctorsexcise.com/journal/borg/htm

Brink, T.L., Yesavage, J.A., Lum, O., Heersema, P., Adey, M.B., and Rose, T.L. (1982) Screening Tests for Geriatric Depression. *Clinical Gerontologist, 1,* 37–44.

Charlesworth, R. (2003). *Understanding Child Development.* Thomson Delmar Learning. Clifton Park, NY.

Christiansen, C., Baum, M.C., and Bass-Haugen, J. (Eds.). (2005). *Occupational Therapy: Performance, Participation, and Well-being.* Slack, Inc. Thorofare, NJ.

Executive Functions. Encyclopedia of Mind Disorders. (2007). Retrieved April 25, 2009, from http://www.minddisorders.com/Del-Fi/Executive-function.html

Falls Assessment Kits: Physiological Profile Assessment Tests. Retrieved November 23, 2009, from www.powmri.edu.au/FBRG using the search engine Google and key words "fall prevention programs."

Feder, G., Cryer, C., Donovan, S., and Carter, Y. (2000). Guidelines for the Prevention of Falls in People over 65. *BMJ, 321,* 1007–1011.

Fiese, B.H., Tomcho, T.J., Douglas, M., Josephs, K., Poltrock, S., and Baker, T. (2002). A Review of 50 Years of Research on Naturally Occurring Family Routines and Rituals: Cause for Celebration? *Journal of Family Psychology, 16*, 381–390.

Fisher, A. (2006). Overview of Performance Skills and Client Factors, in *Pedretti's Occupational Therapy: Practice Skills for Physical Dysfunction*. Editors H. Pendleton and W. Schultz-Krohn. Mosby/Elsevier. St. Louis, MO.

Folstein, M., Folstein, S.E., and McHugh, P.R. (1975). "Mini-Mental State": A Practical Method for Grading the Cognitive State of Patients for the Clinician. *Journal of Psychiatric Research, 12*(3), 189–198.

Foreman, M.D., and Grabowski, R. (1992). Diagnostic Dilemma: Cognitive Impairment in the Elderly. *Journal of Gerontological Nursing, 18*, 5–12.

Foreman, M.D., Fletcher, K., Mion, L.C., and Simon, L. (1996). Assessing Cognitive Function. *Geriatric Nursing, 17*, 228–233.

Fuhrer, M.J. (Ed.). (1987). *Rehabilitation Outcomes Analysis and Measurement*. Brookes. Baltimore, MD.

Hinojosa, J., and Kramer, P. (1997). Fundamental Concepts of Occupational Therapy: Occupation, Purposeful Activity, and Function. *American Journal of Occupational Therapy, 51*, 864–866.

Hofmann, Ashley Opp. (2008). Preventing Falls with Occupational Therapy. AOTA. Bethesda, MD.

James, A.B. (2008). Restoring the Role of Independent Person, in *Occupational Therapy for Physical Dysfunction* (6th Ed.). Editors Mary Vining Radomski and Catherine A. Trombly Latham. Wolters Kluwer/Lippincott Williams & Wilkins. Baltimore, MD.

Kramer, S., McGonigel, M., and Kaufmann, R. (1991). Developing the IFSP: Outcomes, Strategies, Activities, and Services, in *Guidelines and Recommended Practices for the Individualized Family Service Plan*. Editors M. McGonigel, R. Kaufmann, and B. Johnson. Association for the Care of Children's Health. Bethesda, MD.

Law, M., Cooper, B., Strong, S., Stewart, D., Rigby, P., and Letts, L. (1996). Person-Environment-Occupation Model: A Transactive Approach to Occupational Performance. *Canadian Journal of Occupational Therapy, 63*, 9–23.

Maher, C., and Bear-Lehman, J. (2008). Orthopaedic Conditions, in *Occupational Therapy for Physical Dysfunction* (6th Ed.). Editors Mary Vining Radomski and Catherine A. Trombly Latham. Wolters Kluwer/Lippincott Williams & Wilkins. Baltimore, MD.

Mosey, A.C. (1996). Applied Scientific Inquiry in the Health Professions: An Epistemological Orientation—Second Edition. AOTA. Bethesda, MD.

Nurit, W., and Michel, A.B. (2003). Rest: A Qualitative Exploration of the Phenomenon. *Occupational Therapy International, 10*, 227–238.

O'Sullivan, S.B., and Schmitz, T.J. (2007). *Physical Rehabilitation* (5th Ed.). F.A. Davis Company. Philadelphia, PA.

Parham, L.D., and Fazio, L.S. (Eds.). (1997). *Play in Occupational Therapy for Children*. Mosby. St. Louis, MO.

Perry, J. (1992). *Gait Analysis: Normal and Pathological Functions*. Slack, Inc. Thorofare, NJ.

Perry, J., Garrett, M., Gronley, J.K., and Mulroy, S.J. (1995). Classification of Walking Handicap in the Stroke Population. *Stroke, 26,* 982–989.

Pessina, M.A., and Orroth, A.C. (2008). Burn Injuries, in *Occupational Therapy for Physical Dysfunction* (6th Ed.). Editors Mary Vining Radomski and Catherine A. Trombly Latham. Wolters Kluwer/Lippincott Williams & Wilkins. Baltimore, MD.

Richard, R.L., and Ward, R.S. (2007). Burns, in *Physical Rehabilitation* (5th Ed.). Editors Susan B. O'Sullivan and Thomas J. Schmitz. F.A. Davis. Philadelphia, PA.

Rogers, J.C., and Holm, M.B. (1994). Assessment of Self-care, in *Functional Performance in Older Adults.* Editors B.R. Bonder and M.B. Wagner. F.A. Davis. Philadelphia, PA.

Segal, R. (2004). Family Routines and Rituals: A Context for Occupational Therapy Interventions. *American Journal of Occupational Therapy, 58,* 499–508.

Sheikh, J.I., and Yesavage, J.A. (1986). Geriatric Depression Scale (GDS): Recent Evidence and Development of a Shorter Version, in *Clinical Gerontology: A Guide to Assessment and Intervention,* 165–173. Editor T.L. Brink. Haworth Press. Binghamton, NY.

Sheikh, J.I., Yesavage, J.A., Brooks, J.O., III, Friedman, L.F., Gratzinger, P. Hill, R.D., Zadeik, A., and Crook, T. (1991). Proposed Factor Structure of the Geriatric Depression Scale. *International Psychogeriatrics, 3,* 23–28.

Sladyk, K. (2005). Documentation, in *Ryan's Occupational Therapy Assistant: Principles, Practice Issues, and Techniques* (4th Ed.). Editors Karen Sladyk and Emeritus Sally E. Ryan. Slack, Inc. Thorofare, NJ.

Sleep. (2007). The Free Dictionary. Retrieved March 16, 2009, from http://freedictionary.org

Sullivan, T., Smith, J., Kermode, J., McIver, E., and Courtemanche, D.J. (1990). Rating the Burn Scar. *Journal of Burn Care and Rehabilitation, 3,* 256–260.

Tecklin, J.S. (2007). *Pediatric Physical Therapy* (4th Ed.). Wolters Kluwer/Lippincott, Williams, & Wilkins. Baltimore, MD.

Uniform Data System for Medical Rehabilitation. (1996). Guide for the Uniform Data Set for Medical Rehabilitation (including the FIM instrument). UDS. Buffalo, NY.

World Health Organization. (2001). International Classification of Functioning, Disability, and Health (ICF). WHO. Geneva.

Wikipedia. Glasgow Coma Scale. (2009). Retrieved March 29, 2009, from http://en.wikipedia.org/wiki/Glasgow_Coma_Scale

Yesavage, J.A. Long Form of the Geriatric Depression Scale. http://www.stanford.edu/~yesavage/GDS.english.long.html

Yesavage, J.A. Short Form of the Geriatric Depression Scale. http://www.stanford.edu/~yesavage/GDS.english.short.html

Yesavage, J.A., Brink, T.L., Rose, T.L., Lum, O., Huang, V., Adey, M.B., and Leirer, V.O. (1983). Development and Validation of a Geriatric Depression Screening Scale: A Preliminary Report. *Journal of Psychiatric Research, 17,* 37–49.

Index

abdominal fullness, 229
abilities and deficits
    autism, 147
    back fusion, 7–8
    brain injury, 65, 179, 222
    bulimia nervosa, 234
    burn patient, 93–94
    CABG, 53–54
    elderly person, 123
    hip replacement, 75–76
    knee surgery, 102–103
    multiple system failure, 16
    paranoid schizophrenia, 239
    rollover crash victim, 84
    spinal cord injuries, 7–8, 33, 65, 113, 198–199
    stroke patient, 179
activities of daily living
    back fusion, 5–6
    bilateral knee osteoarthritis, 98–100
    brain and spinal cord injury, 29–32
    burn patient, 90–91
    CABG, 12–14, 49–51
    coronary artery bypass graft, 12–14, 49–51
    hip replacement, 73–74
    knee replacement, 41–42
    multiple system failure, 20–21
    spinal cord and brain injuries, 29–32, 59–62, 109–111
adolescent caucasian girl, vehicle crash, 79–86
AIS. *See* Asia Impairment Scale
ALF. *See* assisted living facility
Alzheimer's disease, primary caregiver, 47
American Indian, male. *See* multiple system failure
American Spinal Injury Association (ASIA)
    impairment scale, 27, 29
ASIA. *See* American Spinal Injury Association
Asia Impairment Scale (AIS), 27, 29, 109
assisted living facility (ALF), 48
autism
    abilities, 147
    activities of daily living, 144–145
    bilateral knee osteoarthritis, 102
    communication skills, 146
    consultation, 148
    cultural context, 146–147
    deficits, 147

    discharge, 148
    education, 145, 149
    elementary-school-aged child, 143–144
    habits and routines, 146
    institute, 151–152
    intervention, 147–149
    leisure, 145
    motor skills, 146
    process skills, 146
    routines, 146
    social participation, 145

back fusion
    ability and deficit synthesis, 7–8
    activities of daily living, 5–6
    balance, 119
    consultation process, 9
    contextual factors, 7
    discharge needs, 8
    education process, 9
    home management, 6
    intervention implementation, 8–9
    objective and measurable goals, 8
    working woman, 3–9
Baghdad, Iraq, 217
bathing, 12
bilateral knee osteoarthritis
    activities of daily living, 98–100
    communication skills, 101
    contextual factors, 102
    habits, 101–102
    intervention plan and implementation, 103–104
    motor skills, 100–110
    occupational performance, 102–103
    occupational profile, 97–98
    process skills, 101
    routines, 102
bladder management, 13
bowel management, 13
brain injury, 107–109
    activities of daily living, 29–32
    middle-age male, 127
    mild, 127, 191
    occupational profile, 29
    social participation, 31

spinal cord and, 57–59
spinal cord injury and, 27
brain
areas of function, 174*f*
parts, 174*f*
sectional view, 98*f*
bulimia nervosa
abilities and deficits, 234
activities of daily living, 231–232
affects, 230*f*
contextual factors, 234
education, 232
intervention, 234–236
leisure, 232
occupational profile and performance, 231, 234
performance skills, 233
social participation, 233
teenager, 229
work, 232
burn care, inpatient rehabilitation, 89
burn patient
abilities, 93–94
activities of daily living, 90–91
communication skills, 93
contextual factors, 93
deficits, 93–94
discharge, 94
interaction skills, 93
intervention, 94–96
motor skills, 92
partial-thickness, 89
pediatric treatment, burns, 89–96
play and leisure, 91
profile
rule of nines, 90*f*
sensation, 92
skin characteristics, 92
social participation, 91
treatment, 89–96

CABG. *See* coronary artery bypass graft
case management (CM), 4
central nervous system, spinal nerves, posterior
view, 28*f*
certified occupational therapy assistant (COTA),
215–216
chest tube drain, 27
CM. *See* case management
communication and interaction skills, spinal cord and
brain injuries, 32
computed tomography (CT), 229
contextual factors
back fusion, 7
bilateral knee osteoarthritis, 102
bulimia nervosa, 234
burn patient, 93
coronary bypass graft, 52–53
Guillain-Barré syndrome, 159
hand therapy, 187

hip replacement, 75
knee replacement, 43
multiple system failure, 23
spinal cord injuries, 64, 134, 198
traumatic brain injury, 221–222
coordination, spinal cord and brain injuries, 32
coronary artery bypass graft (CABG), 15–18
activities of daily living, bathing, 12–14, 49–51
acute care elderly person, 11
bladder management, 49
bowel management, 49
contextual factors, 52–53
discharge, 54
dressing, 49
education, 51
habits, 52
intervention implementation, 54–55
intervention plan, 53
leisure, 51
mobility, 49
motor skills, 51–52
occupational performance, 53
occupational profile, 47–49
process skills, 52
roles, 52
routines, 52
sexual activity, 49–50
social participation, 51
treatment, 47
work, 51
COTA. *See* certified occupational therapy assistant
CT. *See* computed tomography
cultural context, CABG, 15–16

diabetes mellitus (DM), 110
dieting obsession, 231
DM. *See* diabetes mellitus
dressing, 13
hip replacement, 73
driving
in-vehicle testing, 167–169
pre-vehicle testing, 164–167
restrictions, 170–171
road performance, 168–169
dyspnea, 229

education, CABA, 14
educational participation, back fusion, 6
elderly person
activities of daily living, 120–121
driving ability, 163–164
fall prevention, 119
intervention implementation, 124–125
intervention plan, 123–124
motor skills, 122
occupational performance, 123
social participation, 121
emergency responses, 14
energy, spinal cord and brain injuries, 32

falling
    fear of, 119
    history of, 119
    prevention, 141–142
femur, anterior and posterior views, 72*f*
financial management, 14
Foley catheter, 27, 109

GCS. *See* Glascow Coma Scale
Glascow Coma Scale (GCS), 27
Guillain-Barré syndrome, 155
    activities of daily living, 157
    consultation, 161
    contextual factors, 159
    education, 161
    intervention, 160–161
    leisure, 157
    motor skills, 158
    nerve damage, 155
    occupational profile and performance, 157, 159
    process skills, 158
    routines, 159
    social participation, 157
    treatment, 155–162

habits, 43. *See also* routines
    autism, 146
    back fusion and, 7
    bilateral knee osteoarthritis, 102–102
    brain injury, 15
    bulimia nervosa, 233
    CABG, 52
    Guillain-Barre, 159
    hand therapy, 186–187
    knee replacement, 43
    multiple system failure, 23
    paranoid schizophrenia, 242
    psychiatric patient, 242
    sepsis, 23
    spinal cord and brain injuries, 32, 64, 112, 133
    stroke patient, 101–102, 178
    traumatic brain injury, 221
hand therapy, 183–184
    activities of daily living, 184–185
    contextual factors, 187
    discharge, 188
    function, 184
    habits and routines, 186–187
    health management, 185
    intervention, 186–189
    job performance, 185
    leisure, 185
    motor skills, 186
    occupational performance, 187
    process skills, 186
    roles, 186
    social participation, 186
health management, 14
    back fusion, 6

heart, anterior view, 12*f*, 48*f*
Heparin, 57
HHC. *See* home health care
hip replacement
    abilities synthesis, 75–76
    activities of daily living, 73–74
    barriers to occupational performance, 76
    contextual factors, 75
    deficits synthesis, 75–76
    discharge needs and plan, 76
    home management, 74
    intervention plan and implementation, 76–77
    job performance, 74
    leisure participation, 74
    motor skills, 74–75
    process skills, 75
    social participation, 74
Hmong community, 239
home health care (HHC), 28
home management, 14
    back fusion, 6
    hip replacement, 74
HTN. *See* hypertension
hypertension (HTN), 110

IED. *See* improvised explosive device
improvised explosive device (IED), 217
instrumental activities of daily living, spinal cord injury and
    brain injuries, 30–31
intervention plan
    back fusion, 8
    CABG, 16–18
    knee replacement, 44–46
    rollover crash victim, 84–85
    spinal cord and brain injuries, 65–67, 113–115
    spinal cord injury, 33–35
invertebral disc, damage in, 3

knee joint, anterior view, 40*f*
knee replacement
    activities of daily living, 41–42
    contextual factors, 43
    discharge needs, 44
    habits and routines, 43
    intervention, 44–46
    motor skills, 42–43
    occupational performance, 43–44
    occupational profile, 41
    process skills, 43
    role fulfillment, 43
    social participation, 42
    Spanish-speaking woman, 39–40

leisure, 14
    activities, back fusion and, 6
lumbar spinal fusion, 3

magnetic resonance imaging (MRI), 3
mobility, 13
    hip replacement, 73

knee surgery, 99
spinal cord and brain injuries, 32
motorcycle crash, 107–109, 191–193
motor skills
American Indian male, 22
autism, 146
back fusion, 6–7
bilateral knee osteoarthritis, 100–101
brain injury, 31, 111–112, 132–133, 220–221
burn victim, 92
CABG, 15, 51–52
elderly person, 122, 164–167
Guillain-Barré syndrome, 158
hand therapy, 186
hip replacement, 74–75
knee replacement, 42–43
multiple system failure, 22
osteoarthritis, 74–75
paranoid schizophrenia, 242
rollover accident, 82–83
spinal cord injury, 31, 63, 111–112, 132–133, 196–197
stroke, 177
motor vehicle operation, restrictions, 170
MRI. *See* magnetic resonance imaging
multiple system failure, 19–20
abilities and deficits, 23–24
activities of daily living, 20–21
habits and 8, 23
instrumental activities, 21
intervention implementation, 24–25
intervention plan, 24
motor skills, 22
occupational profile, 20
process skills, 23
profile, 19–20
respiratory function, 22
roles, 23
sensation, 22
skin characteristics, 22
social participation, 21–22
multipolar neuron anatomy, 156*f*

nerve injuries, 183–184
nerves
peripheral, 184
spinal cord and, 128, 192*f*
in-vehicle testing, 167–169

occupational performance
bilateral knee osteoarthritis, 102–103
brain injury, 29, 59, 109, 131
bulimia nervosa, 231, 234
CABG, 16
coronary artery disease, 47–49, 53
elderly person, 123
Guillain-Barré, 157, 159
hand therapy, 187
knee replacement, 43–44

multiple system failure, 20
paranoid schizophrenia, 240
post fusion vertebrae, 5
spinal cord injuries, 29, 59, 109, 134, 193, 197
stroke patient, 210
traumatic brain injury, 220
occupational therapy (OT), 4
Operation Iraqi Freedom, 217
Orthodox Jewish male, stroke, 97–98
osteoarthritis, severe right hip, 71–73
osteoposrosis, 119
screening, 141–142
OT. *See* occupational therapy

PAMS. *See* physical agent modalities
paranoid schizophrenia, 239
abilities and deficits, 243
activities of daily living, 240–241
community mobility, 241
contextual factors, 242–243
education, 241
habits and routines, 242
health management, 241
intervention, 243–245
leisure, 241
motor and process skills, 242
occupational profile, 240
process skills, 239–245
roles, 242
social participation, 241–242
work, 241
PE. *See* pulmonary embolism
pediatric treatment, burns, 89–96
peripheral nervous system, axon anatomy, 156*f*
physical agent modalities (PAMS), 216
physical therapy (PT), 4
pneumonia, 27, 57, 127, 191
post spine surgery, 4
posture, spinal cord and brain injuries, 32
process skills
Alzheimers, 52
autism, 146
back fusion, 7
bilateral knee osteoarthritis, 101
brain injuries. *See* spinal cord and brain injuries
bulimia nervosa, 233
burn victims, 93
CABG, 15, 52
Guillain-Barré syndrome, 158
hand therapy, 186
hip replacement, 75
knee replacement, 43
osteoarthritis, 75
osteoporosis, 122
paranoid schizophrenia, 239–245
rollover motor vehicle crash victim, 83
spinal cord and brain injuries, 32, 64, 112, 133, 197
stroke patient, 177
traumatic brain injury, 221

psychiatric treatment
   bulimia, 230
   paranoid schizophrenia, 239–245
PT. *See* physical therapy
pulmonary embolism (PE), 27, 57, 127, 191

rest, 13
right coxal bone, medial view, 72*f*
roles
   back fusion and, 7
   CABG, 15, 52
   hand therapy, 186
   knee replacement, 43
   multiple system failure, 23
   paranoid schizophrenia, 242
   spinal cord and brain injuries, 32, 112, 133
   spinal cord injury, 197–198
rollover motor vehicle crash victim, 79–86
   abilities and deficits, 84
   communication skills, 83
   cultural contexts, 83–84
   discharge needs, 85–86
   education and work, 81–82
   instrumental activities, 81
   intervention plan, 84–85
   leisure and social participation, 82
   motor skills, 82–83
   process skills, 83
   profile, 79–80
routines, 83. *See also* habits
   autism, 146
   back fusion and, 7
   bilateral knee osteoarthritis, 102
   brain injury, 32, 64, 112
   CABG, 15, 52
   hand therapy, 186
   knee replacement, 43
   spinal cord injuries, 64, 197
   traumatic brain injury, 221

safety, 14
sexual activity, 13
shopping, back fusion, 6
skilled nursing facility (SNF), 28
sleep, 13
SNF. *See* skilled nursing facility
social participation, 14–15
   back fusion and, 6
   CABG, 14–15
   stroke patient, 177
spinal cord injury, 29, 59, 107–109, 131, 134
   abilities and deficits, 33, 198–199
   activities of daily living, 193–195
   brain injury and. *See* spinal cord injury, brain injury and
   communication skills, 197
   consultation and education, 34–35
   contextual factors, 198
   contextual influences, 32–33
   discharge needs, 34

   functional mobility, 194
   intervention, 33–35, 199–200
   leisure, 195–196
   motorcycle crash, 191
   motor skills, 196–197
   occupational profile, 193
   process skills, 197
   roles, 197–198
   sleep/rest, 194
   social participation, 196
   traumatic, 193
   work, 195
spinal cord injury, brain injury and, 27, 57–59, 191
   abilities and deficits, 65
   activities of daily living, 29–32, 59–62, 109–111, 129–131
   bowel and bladder management, 109
   communication skills, 64, 112, 133
   complete tetraplegia, 109
   consultation, 136
   contextual factors, 64, 134
   cultural factors, 112
   discharge, 65–66, 135
   education, 62, 111
   habits and routines, 64, 112, 133
   interaction skills, 64, 112
   intervention, 65–67, 113–115, 130, 135–136
   leisure, 62, 131–132
   motor skills, 63, 111–112, 132–133
   nerves, spinal cord and, 58*f*, 128*f*
   occupational performance, 29, 59, 109, 134
   performance, 59–61
   physical factors, 112
   process skills, 64, 112, 133
   roles, 112, 133
   routines, 64
   social participation, 31, 62, 113, 131
   strength and effort, 32
   traumatic, 129
   work, 62, 131
spinal cord, nerves and, 108*f*, 192*f*
stroke patient, 173–174, 203
   abilities, 179
   activities of daily living, 174–175, 203–204
   behind wheel testing, 204–207
   deficits, 179
   discharge needs, 179–180
   driving performance, 203–207
   habits, 178
   instrumental activities, 175–176
   intervention plan and implementation, 179–181, 210–11
   leisure, 176
   motor skills, 177
   occupational performance, 210
   on-the-road performance, 208–209
   Orthodox Jewish male, 97–98
   process skills, 177
   routines, 178
   social participation, 177
   work, 176

tetraplegia, 191
  complete, 109
toileting, 13
  hip replacement, 73
traumatic brain injury
  abilities, 222
  activities of daily living, 218–220
  communication skills, 221
  contextual factors, 221–222
  deficits, 222
  habits, 221
  interaction skills, 221
  intervention, 222–225
  job performance, 220
  leisure, 220
  motor skills, 220–221
  process skills, 221
  routines, 221
  social participation, 220

vertebra anatomy, 4f

Walter Reed Medical Hospital, 217
Warrior Support Triad, 218
Warrior Transition Unit (WTU), phases of care, 218
WTU. See Warrior Transition Unit
work
  back fusion and, 3–9
  bilateral knee osteoarthritis, 102–103
  brain injury, 29, 59, 109, 134
  brain and spinal cord injuries, 62, 131
  bulimia, 232
  CABG, 14, 51
  elderly person, 123
  Guillain-Barré syndrome, 157, 159
  hand therapy, 187
  hip replacement, 74
  knee replacement, 41, 43–44
  multiple system failure, 20
  paranoid schizophrenia, 240
  spinal cord injuries, 29, 59, 62, 109, 131, 134, 193
  stroke patient, 176
  traumatic brain injury, 220